Abstracts of the 65th Congress of the German Society of Neurology

23–26 September 1992   Saarbrücken, FRG

Congress President

K. Schimrigk, Homburg/Saar

Secretary

A. Haass, Homburg/Saar

Advisory Board

T. Brandt, München
H. C. Diener, Essen
A. Haass, Homburg/Saar
W. Hacke, Heidelberg
H. C. Hopf, Mainz
F. Jerusalem, Bonn
E. Klippel, Hünfeld
D. Koch, Magdeburg

D. Kömpf, Lübeck
K. Kunze, Hamburg
B. Neundörfer, Erlangen
H. Przuntek, Bochum
K. Schimrigk, Homburg/Saar
K. Toyka, Würzburg
A. Wagner, Leipzig

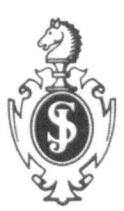

Springer-Verlag Berlin Heidelberg GmbH

ISBN 978-3-662-38797-9   ISBN 978-3-662-39699-5 (eBook)
DOI 10.1007/978-3-662-39699-5

Contents

Platform session I
Ophthalmoneurology

1

The Oculomotor System: Two Goals, Two Modes, Five Systems
D. Kömpf

Eye movements serve vision by placing the image of an object of regard on the fovea of each retina and by preventing slippage of images on the retina. The brain employs two modes of ocular motor control: Fast eye movements (saccades) and smooth (slow) pursuit eye movements (SPEM). Five distinct ocular motor systems are utilized to achieve clear vision. Four of the systems generate conjugate movements (version), one system generates dysjunctive horizontal movements (vergence).

1. Saccades achieve rapid fixation of targets that fall on the extrafoveal retina by moving the eyes at peak velocities up to 700 deg/sec. Quick nystagmus phases are also saccades generated by the same neurons in pons and midbrain. The saccadic system arises mainly from the frontal eye field (FEF, area 8) . The FEF projects directly to the pontine (PPRF, horizontal) and mesodiencephalic (riMLF, vertical) saccadic generating centers, this pathway decussating at the junction of the midbrain and pons. Saccades from the occipital lobe get direct access to the brainstem via the superior colliculus (SC) . There is another third - indirect - pathway through the caudate nucleus, the pars reticulata of the substantia nigra and the SC; this pathway is tonically inhibitory to the SC. The cortex initiates and voluntarily controls saccadic eye movements, the control signals, however, are generated in brainstem supranuclear gaze centers (PPRF, riMLF). Vertical gaze - as a general principle - is mediated by bilateral circuits.

2. Smooth pursuit maintains fixation of slowly moving target. The SPEM-system starts where vision is primarily received (area 17) responding to slippage of an image near the fovea. Axons from the striate cortex project to extrastriate visual areas (middle temporal visual area MT, medio-superior temporal area MST, posterior parietal region) , from here ipsilaterally to the dorsolateral pontine nuclei, then to the flocculus and the dorsal vermis of the cerebellum, then to the oculomotor nuclei: Concept of an ipsilateral parietooccipito-ponto-cerebellar pathway. It is interesting that this pathway unlike the saccadic pathway goes from the brainstem to the cerebellum and then back to the brainstem, whereas the saccadic pathway goes directly from cerebral hemisphere to brainstem.

3. The vestibulo-ocular reflex (VOR) prevents retinal slip during head movements by moving the eyes at the same velocity as the head, but in the opposite direction - the VOR keeps gaze stable relative to the world. Visual cancellation of the VOR occurs when an object is pursued with the head - head and eye moving simultaneously toward the target.

4. Optokinetic smooth eye movements aid vestibular eye movements by stabilizing images on the retina during constant velocity or very low frequency head movements, when the VOR does not function optimally.

5. The vergence system achieves binocular vision by generating dysjunctive eye movements that align the two foveas on an object as it approaches the head; the vergence system is also responsible for maintaining stereoacuity. One of the most complex type of eye movements are the frequently occuring combined vergent-saccadic movements; it is not yet clearly understood how the underlying control signal is generated.

Additionally the cerebellum mediates control of ocular motor systems participating in four major ocular motor functions: a) stabilization of images upon the retina during smooth pursuit, b) regulation of the duration of the vestibulo-ocular responses; the time required for the VOR to discharge is measured by the VOR time constant, c) regulation of saccadic amplitude, and d) repair of ocular dysmetria.

2

THREE-DIMENSIONAL ORGANIZATION OF THE HUMAN OCULOMOTOR SYSTEM

M.Fetter, D.Tweed*, E.Koenig

Neurologische Klinik, Universität Tübingen, Hoppe-Seyler Str. 3, D-7400 Tübingen, Germany and *Department of Physiology, University of Western Ontario, London, Canada

Three-dimensional (3-D) eye movements during steady fixation and saccades are governed by a powerful strategy which confines all possible 3-D eye positions to a 2-D subspace, i.e. angular position vectors of the eye all lie in a single plane (Listing's law) [1,2]. A geometric consequence of this law is that eye velocity vectors also lie in distinct planes which are dependent on eye position. In general, the velocity plane should always be rotated in the same direction as the eye, but only half as far (tilt factor 0.5) [2]. This study was designed to test whether other oculomotor subsystems like smooth pursuit and the optokinetic (OKR) and vestibuloocular reflexes (VOR) also obey this law.

Using the magnetic search coil technique, we recorded 3-D eye position during smooth pursuit (8 subjects), OKR (3 subjects) and VOR (6 subjects). For all experiments subjects were firmly seated in a computer-controlled chair which could be moved about any axis in space via a gimbal system with two motor-driven axes. The subject was surrounded by an opaque fiberglass sphere of radius 1m. During saccade and pursuit experiments, the subject maintained fixation on a red laser light spot projected onto the inner surface of the sphere. The laser could be pointed in any direction within about 30° of straight ahead by two computer-controlled mirrors. We use the angular position vector (actually the vector part of the eye position "quaternion") and the angular velocity vector for describing eye position and velocity.

We showed for any given target motion that during smooth pursuit, as during saccades and fixation, the rotation axis of the eye does indeed depend on the direction of the gaze line (or target), and that the velocity vectors tilt, on average, only about half as far as the gaze line (average tilt factor 0.5) [3]. This arrangement means that pursuit, saccades and fixation can follow one another in quick succession without carrying the eye position vector out of the common (Listing's) eye position plane.

In contrast, for perfect full-field image stabilization during OKR and VOR, the axis of eye rotation should theoretically be independent of the eye position; e.g. for the VOR, eye velocity should be equal and opposite to head velocity, regardless of eye position (tilt factor 0). For the OKR studies, the subjects tracked a field of projected light spots rotating about various axes (horizontal, vertical, torsional) with a constant velocity of 60°/s. For VOR, the subjects were rotated about body-vertical, naso-occipital, and interaural axes in complete darkness sinusoidally at 0.3 Hz with an amplitude of ± 20° and a maximum speed of 37°/s.

Unlike smooth pursuit the OKR and VOR show a pattern of position dependence lying about halfway between the optimal (no dependence) and that characteristic of Listing's law (average tilt factors: OKR = 0.35, VOR = 0.26). This behaviour may be a compromise aimed at restricting ocular torsion but is incompatible with optimal retinal image stabilization. We postulate that Listing's law is not primarily a function of orbital mechanics. The mechanisms responsible for the law must be assigned to the brain. It would seem reasonable to give the computational job of implementing Listing's law to neural networks, which could then be put at the service of only those eye movement systems requiring them. The site of these networks remains to further studies.

References

1. Helmholtz H von (1867) Handbuch der Physiologischen Optik, 1st edn, Vol.3, Voss, Hamburg
2. Tweed D, Vilis T (1990) Geometric relations of eye position and veloctiy vectors during saccades. Vision Res. 30, 111-127
3. Tweed D, Fetter M, Andreadaki S, Koenig E, Dichgans J (1992) Three-dimensional properties of human pursuit eye movements. Vision Res (in press)

This study was supported by the Deutsche Forschungsgemeinschaft, SFB 307, A2. D.T. was a fellow of the Medical Research Council of Canada.

3

The neuronal representation of smooth-pursuit eye movements: implications for neurological diagnosis
P. Thier and J. Dichgans, Department of Neurology, Tübingen, Germany.

Smooth-pursuit eye movements are executed by man and non-human primates in order to minimize slip of the retinal image of a moving visual target. Converging evidence based on work on monkeys and on studies of the oculomotor consequences of lesions in humans (for review, conf. to 1,2,3) suggests a first sketch of the circuitry underlying smooth-pursuit eye movements in man.

In order to minimize retinal target slip, information on the retinal displacement of the target image has to be derived. This is accomplished by a cortical area, termed *MT* in monkeys, which in humans seems to comprise parts of areas 19, 37 and 38. Lesions affecting this or earlier parts of the visual system will cause a contralateral scotoma for motion independent of its direction (the "retinal" pursuit deficit). A subsequent stage of processing is represented by *area MSTl* of monkeys, whose human homologue is probably localized at the junction of the occipital, temporal and parietal lobes. Lesions of this part of the brain cause a non-retinal deficit which, independent of the localization of the target image on the retina, leads to impairment of smooth-pursuit to the ipsilateral side (the so-called "motor" pursuit deficit). Pursuit-related signals originating from the cortical areas mentioned are forwarded to lobuli VI-IX of the *cerebellar vermis* by way of the *dorsolateral* part of the *pontine nucleus*. Lesions of this cortico-ponto-cerebellar pathway at various levels including the internal capsule next to the thalamus, the dorsolateral pons and the cerebellar vermis have been shown to cause pursuit deficits which resemble those due to parietooccipital lesions. Although the exact route linking the pursuit-related parts of the cerebellar vermis with the final eye movement effector in the oculomotor nuclei is still controversial, it is clear from single-unit recordings in monkeys that it must involve the *vestibular nuclei* as a final premotor element. Our recent observation of a contralateral pursuit-deficit in man following a cancerous lesion of large parts of the vestibular nuclei is in accordance with this view. Several lines of evidence suggest that the posterior vermis, the major cerebellar target of the cortico-ponto-cerebellar projection described, subserves a more general function contributing to all forms of voluntary eye movements. In other words the simplistic notion of a division of labour between first the *posterior vermis* and second the *flocculus* and *ventral paraflocculus*, the former thought to be responsible for saccades and the latter for pursuit, is no longer tenable. Why there is need for two distinct regions in the cerebellum dealing with pursuit-related information is one of many unanswered questions which will have to be tackled by future research. Other questions relate to the role of structures outside the direct parietooccipito-ponto-cerebellar pathway outlined here, including the *frontal eye fields*, the *accessory optic system* and the *NRTP* (=N. retic. tegm. pontis).

[1] *Leigh, RJ* (1989) The control of ocular pursuit movements. Revue Neurol. 145: 605-612

[2] *Newsome, WT and Wurtz, RH* (1988) Probing visual cortical function with discrete chemical lesions. TINS 11: 394-399

[3] *Thier, P, Bachor, A, Koenig, E, Dichgans, J* (1991) Selective impariment of smooth-pursuit eye movements due to an ischemic lesion of the basal pons. Annals of Neurol. 29: 443-448

Supported by DFG SFB 307-A1

4

EYE-HEAD COORDINATION IN PATIENTS WITH CHRONIC BILATERAL VESTIBULAR LOSS
Th. Mergner, Ch. Maurer, W. Becker
Neurologie Freiburg, Sektion Neurophysiologie Ulm

Gaze saccades normally consist of an eye saccade in combination with a head saccade. Usually the head saccade starts later and lasts longer than the eye saccade, so that the head is still moving while the eyes already reached target. During the ongoing head movement the eyes are counter-rotated in the orbit in order to keep gaze on the target. Earlier studies suggested that the vestibulo-ocular reflex (VOR) plays a major role in the control of this eye-head coordination. We investigated this mechanism by comparing horizontal eye-head saccades of six normal subjects (Ns) to those of six patients with chronic bilateral vestibular loss (Ps). Saccades were performed in a head-fixed condition (target displacements, 5-60°) and in a head-free condition (10-120°). They were analyzed separately for centrifugal, centripetal, and symmetrical (about primary position) target displacements.

Results. Head-fixed condition: Amplitude, duration, and peak velocity of eye saccades in Ps were similar to those in Ns, whereas eye latency was, on the average, longer in Ps by approximately 40 msec.

Head-free condition: Latency of eye saccades again was longer in Ps by 40 msec, and latency of head saccades was longer by 80 msec. Furthermore, amplitude and peak velocity of head saccades in Ps were only half of those of Ns, and head duration was prolonged in Ps. On the other hand, eye saccades in Ps had larger amplitudes, longer durations, and higher peak velocities than in Ns. As a consequence, the gaze saccades in Ps had approximately the same accuracy as in Ns, but reached target slightly later (see Fig. 1).

Discussion. We interpret the abnormally late and small head saccades in Ps as a change in eye-head strategy which Ps use to reduce interference of their eye saccade by the head movement. Apparently, non-vestibular (visual, neck proprioceptive, preprogrammed) mechanisms cannot fully take over the role which the VOR normally plays for eye-head coordination during gaze saccades.

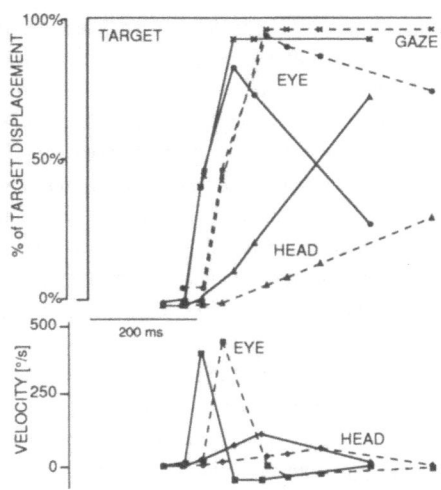

Fig. 1. Target, gaze, eye, and head position as well as eye and head velocity as a function of time in Ns (full lines) and Ps (dashed lines). Averages across distinct measuring points for all 5-60 ° centrifugal saccades.

5

THE CONTRIBUTION OF OTOLITH STIMULATION TO VESTIBULAR NYSTAGMUS IN HUMANS

E. Koenig, M. Fetter, D. Tweed[*], D. Fischer, H. Misslisch. Neurologische Klinik, Universität Tübingen, D-7400 Tübingen, Germany; [*]Department of Physiology, University of Western Ontario, London, Canada.

Vestibular nystagmus is traditionally tested by rotating the subject around an earth-vertical axis (i.e. mainly by stimulating the horizontal semicircular canals) and is characterized by its gain and the time constant of its decline. In order to test the vertical semicircular canals and otoliths as well, a new multiaxis rotating chair was constructed which spins a human subject around any axis with respect to the body and with respect to gravity. Rotations around an earth-horizontal axis lead to dynamic otolith stimulation in addition to the semicircular canal stimulus.

To quantify the vestibulo-ocular reflex (VOR) in humans during rotations around the three major body axes with and without dynamic otolith stimulation, 6 normal subjects were accelerated in total darkness within 1 second to a final velocity of 150°/s. After 30 s of constant-velocity rotation, subjects were decelerated within 1 s to a standstill. The rotation axis ran through the center of the head. Rotations were performed in both directions around each of the yaw, pitch and roll axes of the head, with the axis earth-vertical or earth-horizontal, for a total of 12 rotations/subject. Horizontal, vertical and torsional eye movements were recorded with the search coil technique.

The 3-dimensional description of the VOR requires the use of a 3 x 3 matrix describing the dependence of all 3 components of eye velocity on all 3 components of head velocity). The 3 x 3 matrix showed only minimal components of eye movements orthogonal to the stimulation axis. Gains during the first second of constant-velocity stimulation were rather low and showed no difference between earth-vertical and earth-horizontal rotation. Gains were highest for rotation in yaw (average horizontal VOR gain: -.37), smaller in pitch (vertical VOR: -.25) and smallest in roll (torsional VOR: -.2). Whereas horizontal and torsional VOR were directionally symmetric (right versus left, clockwise versus counterclockwise), the vertical VOR was considerably stronger for backward head rotation (VOR slow phase downward: gain = -.36) compared to forward head rotation (VOR slow phase upwards: gain = -.11) during earth-vertical stimulation (lying on the side). This asymmetry of the vertical VOR was smaller during earth-horizontal rotation (i.e. pitch in the upright body position with dynamic otolith stimulation by gravity): gain for pitch backward = -.30, for forward = -.20.

As known from earlier experiments, vestibular nystagmus does not decline to 0 with off-vertical rotation but to a low velocity around which the eye velocity undulates in synchrony with body rotation in space. For this reason, time constants were not measured for earth-horizontal rotation. For earth-vertical rotation, time constants were longest for horizontal VOR (10.2 s) and shorter for the vertical and torsional VOR (5.0 s, 5.5 s). Whereas the time constants of horizontal and torsional VOR were again symmetrical, the time constant of the vertical VOR elicited by backward head movements was slightly longer (5.4 s) than that for downward head movements (4.7 s).

In summary, the human VOR is mainly driven by the semicircular canals at the onset of constant-velocity stimulation. There is no significant difference between earth-horizontal and earth-vertical rotation for horizontal and torsional VOR. Dynamic otolith stimulation diminishes the asymmetry of the vertical VOR and leads to continuous nystagmus as long as the rotation lasts.

This study was supported by the Deutsche Forschungsgemeinschaft grant SFB 307, A2. D. Tweed was a Fellow of the Medical Research Council of Canada.

6

CYTOKINE STUDIES IN OPTIC NEURITIS.

Hans-Peter Hartung and Klaus V. Toyka, MS Clinical Research Group, Department of Neurology, University of Würzburg

Cytokines are mediators that are generated and released in the course of an immune response. They orchestrate the actions of immunocompetent cells. To elucidate immune mechanisms in the pathogenesis of optic neuritis we looked at serum cytokine levels in 46 patients who presented with acute monocular ON. In 21 patients clinical examination, evoked potential studies and MRI revealed multiple brain lesions. Fifty-five patients with other neurological diseases and 26 healthy volunteers served as controls. Serum concentrations of IL-1ß, IL-2, sIL-2R, TNF-α, and IL-6 were measured by ELISA. We found in 8 of 25 patients with isolated ON elevated concentrations of IL-2 and sIL-2R as well as increased IL-6 concentrations. Eleven of 21 patients with additional CNS lesions had increased IL-2 and sIL-2R levels while 8 of 21 had increased IL-6 lebels. IL-1 and TNF-α were not detected. Taken together, these results provide evidence for systemic T- and B-cell activation in a proportion of patients with optic neuritis.

7

DISORDERS OF COLOUR PERCEPTION IN PARKINSON'S DISEASE

Th.Büttner, W.Kuhn, P,Klotz, R.Steinberg, M.Langkafel, H.Przuntek
Department of Neurology, Ruhr-University Bochum, St.Josef-Hospital, Bochum, Germany

Introduction:
Dysfunctions of the visual system in Parkinson's disease (PD) could be proven by alterations in contrast sensitivity and delayed latencies of visual evoked potentials. However, colour perception has to our knowledge never been studied in Parkinsonians. We observed a patient with a malignant neuroleptic syndrome who under the treatment with lisuride mispercepted a red point as a red line. After dosage reduction of lisuride this misperception vanished.
Additionally, coloured hallucinations were a quite frequent phenomenon of our patients with PD under treatment with lisuride. We suppose that those phenomena could be interpreted as a consequence of disturbed spatial acuicy of colour perception. We therefore developed a computer-aided method to measure the perception of colour fusion.

Patients and methods:
A colour computer monitor system presents a horizontal monochromatic coloured bar with a temporal frequency of 6/s. The bar is subdivided into 60 segments which enlarge discontinually during the experiment and confluence to a homogenous bar within 10 seconds. As soon as the patient percepts a homogenous unsegmented bar he tells the investigator to stop the experiment. The computer system transforms the latencies till subjective fusion of the segments into points from 0 to 100. We present the colours red, green, yellow and blue, a bright and a dark version respectively. Additionally a black and a white stimulus are presented to estimate the achromatic fusion time. The study comprises 83 patients with PD with an average age of 65,3 +/- 9,6 years (range 47 - 84 years). Among this sample are 15 patients who didn't got any treatment before (de novo-patients). The control group consists of 60 probands with an average age of 48,5 +/- 15,4 years (range 27 - 80 years).

Results:
Patients with PD were characterized by a shortened colour fusion time. This phenomenon was observed for each tested colour, but it was statistically significant for the darkgreen stimulus. The fusion time for chromatic stimuli depended on the severity ($p < 0,001$ for the darkgreen stimulus) and the duration of PD. The colour fusion time of de novo patients differed slightly from that of treated patients. The analysis of patients in early disease-stages shows that the treated population had a longer colour fusion latency than the de novo-patients. Patients on treatment with bromocriptine had a normalized fusion time compared to those without any dopaminergic treatment. On the contrary those patients who got lisuride as a dopamine agonist had a shortened colour fusion latency

Discussion:
Experimental neurophysiological examinations of the last few years pointed out that the colour perception is performed in a specialized neuronal system distinct from the achromatic visual system. The spatial solution of the chromatic system is coarse in comparison with the achromatic system. This difference in spatial acuicy explains a shortened subjective fusion of coloured stimuli as compared with achromatic stimuli even in our control group. However, this physiological phenomenon was considerably intensified in PD. We suppose that the phenomenon is related to dopamine deficiency because the misperception couldn't be demonstrated in treated patients in early stages of the disease wheras it was present in de novo patients. The opposite effects of lisuride and bromocriptine on colour fusion might be due to the principle pharmacological difference of both drugs.

8

RECOVERY CYCLE OF THE BLINK REFLEX IN BLEPHAROSPASM

Wöbker G, Cramer S, Ferbert A
Department of Neurology, RWTH Aachen, 5100 Aachen, FRG

The neurological basis of blepharospasm is still not fully understood. Indirect arguments favour an organic origin and the condition has been classified as one type of torsion dystonia (Marsden 1976). Nevertheless, direct evidence for this hypothesis is still scarce and some authors still maintain that the condition might be psychogenic. This controversy is in part caused by a lack of abnormal findings in imaging or neurophysiological tests. Earlier studies have found abnormalities of the electrically elicited blink reflex in patients with blepharospasm (Berardelli et al. 1985, Tolosa et al. 1988). These authors found an increase of the R1-component and a prolongation and amplitude increase of the R2-component. However, these parameters are quite variable even in healthy subjects and are therefore of little help for the diagnosis in a single patient.
We investigated 9 patients aged 46 to 72 years with clinical signs of blepharospasm. One patient had torticollis, a second patient had oropharyngeal dystonia in addition. The blink reflex was elicited by bipolar stimulation of the supraorbital nerve with a stimulus intensity of 19 to 23 mA. The EMG of the orbicularis oculi muscle (OOM) was recorded with Ag/AgCl surface electrodes placed over the lower and lateral part of the OOM. Double stimuli were applied with an interstimulus interval (ISI) of 100 and 150 ms. In four patients ISI of 300 and 500 ms were tested in addition. Three stimuli were applied per condition. Onset latency of R1 and R2 and duration of R2 were measured as well as maximal peak to peak amplitudes. Results were compared with those of 15 normal controls aged 30 to 67 years.
Latencies of R1- and R2-components were normal in all patients. However, the R2-component was prolonged in patients. Three patients showed contralateral R1-components which could not be found in our controls. Upon double stimulation the R2-component to the second stimulus was inhibited by 80 to 100% at an ISI of 100 ms in normals. In 6 patients this inhibition was markly reduced and in two patients it was normal. The 9th patients showed an increase of the baseline EMG activity of long duration upon the second stimulus. In order to clarify whether involuntary contraction in patients would itself influence the inhibition we stimulated two normal subjects with preinnervation of the OOM of various degrees. The second R2-component was somewhat less inhibited compared to the relaxed state. However, it was still clearly more inhibited than in patients. These findings are in keeping with the hypothesis of disturbed brain stem inhibitory interneurons or with dysfunction of descending pathways from the basal ganglia upon the brain stem nuclei in blepharospasm. From the diagnostic point of view, the blink reflex with double stimuli is a valuable method for the diagnosis of blepharospasm. The blink reflex to single stimuli, while abnormal in a group of patients, does not give results clear enough to make a diagnosis in a single patient.

References:
Berardelli A, Rothwell JC, Day BL, Marsden CD (1985) Pathophysiology of blepharospasm and oromandibular dystonia. Brain 108: 593-608

Marsden CD (1976) Blepharospasm-oromandibular dystonia syndrome (Brueghel's syndrome): A variant of adult-onset torsion dystonia? J. Neurol. Neurosurg. Psychiatr. 39: 1204-1209

Tolosa E, Montserrat L, Bayes A (1988) Blink reflex studies in focal dystonias: Enhanced excitability of brainstem interneurons in cranial dystonia and spasmodic torticollis. Movement Disorders 3: 61-69

9

Blepharospasm as major symptom in Myasthenia gravis

A. Konstanzer A.- O. Ceballos-Baumann, M. Kornhuber, J. Dressnandt, and B. Conrad
Department of Neurology, Technical University Munich

Introduction:
This study reports about 5 patients applying for Botulinum-Toxin (Botox) treatment because of blepharospasm. Careful clinical examination however, revealed additional symptoms which finally led to the diagnosis of Myasthenia gravis.

Patients (see Table 1):
Three females and two males (62 - 72 years, mean age 69,2 y.) with a history of blepharospasm for a mean of 2.8 years were examined. Two (no. 1, 5) had treatment with Botox earlier without success (no. 1) or with severe side effects (worsening of ptosis no. 5).

Additional symptoms (see Table 2):
Double vision with diurnal fluctuations, ptosis, bulbar and generalized weakness after exertion led to the final diagnosis of Myasthenia gravis. The clinical staging according to the Osserman scale was grade I in patients no. 1 and 5, IIa or b in patients no. 2,3,4. Acetylcholin-receptor anti-bodies were positive in two patients (no.3,4).

Therapy:
Four patients were successfully treated with pyridostigmin and corticosteroids (no. 1,2,3,4). Patient no.5 preferred Botox injections of low dose which had moderate effect without side effects.

Discussion:
Since the treatment with Botox injections was successfully introduced in the therapy of blepharospasm, a large number of patients applies for this therapy. Careful clinical examination can exclude severe diseases like Myasthenia gravis. The clinical examination of the patient should contain inspection of the eye to exclude double vision after exertion and ptosis. Additionally, diurnal fluctuations of muscle strenght and bulbar symptoms should be noted.
The reason for exessive eye lid contractions due to Myasthenia gravis can only be speculated upon:
- constant irritation of the cornea by a latent ptosis similar to the lid twitch response
- contractions are meant to increase maximally the level of acetylcholine available to the postsynaptic receptors in order to avoid ptosis and double vision
- a consequence of high innervation levels of the periorbital muscles showing abrupt break down of innervation.

Table 1:
List of patients

No.	age	gender	duration	symptoms
1:	72	male	12 ys.	BPS, diplopia, ptosis
2:	72	female	1 y.	BPS, diplopia
3:	68	female	4 y.	BPS, bulbar weakness
4:	72	female	4 y.	BPS, diplopia, ptosis
5:	62	male	4 y.	BPS, diplopia

Legend:
BPS: blepharospasm

Table 2:
Additional symptoms

Pat. No.	1	2	3	4	5
Osserman grade	I	IIb	IIa	IIb	I
Thymoma	-	-	-	-	-
ACH R AB	-	-	+	+	-
Antinuclear AB	-	-	-	+	-
Smooth MF AB	+	-	-	-	-
Striated MF AB	-	-	+	+	-
Thyreoid AB	+	-	-	+	-
Parietal cell AB	-	-	-	+	-
Tensilon test	+	-	+	+	-
Pyridostigmin	+	+	+	+	-
Corticosteroids	-	+	+	+	-
Botox	-	-	-	-	+

Legend:
AB: antibody
MF: muscle fibre

10

BOTULINUM TOXIN FOR CERVICAL DYSTONIA: PROBLEMS OF ASSESSMENT AND QUANTIFICATION OF THERAPEUTIC EFFECTS.

F.Erbguth, M.-J.Hilz, K.-D.Kilian, Th.Rechlin, D.Claus, B.Neundörfer. Dpt. of Neurology; University Hospital; Erlangen/Germany

Since 1988 120 patients with different types of cervical dystonia have received local injections with Botulinum toxin A (Porton Down; "Dysport^R"). Corresponding to other studies 97 patients (=81%) reported a substantial benefit (more than 50% improvement) after the first course of injections (1-3 injections). Nevertheless it should be pointed out that assessment and control of the therapeutic efficacy and the clinical course is difficult during follow-up. There is a lack of instrumental quantification devices. Most studies don't mention these methodical problems. With the example of our study we shall discuss the difficulties in assessing and quantifying therapeutic effects in patients with cervical dystonia:

1. Placebo-controlled studies are of questionable value. The BOTOX induced atrophy of the hyperactive and hypertrophic sternocleidomastoid muscle makes the verum clearly distinguishable from the placebo. So the intended objectivity cannot be achieved. This visible difference before and after therapy also affects the objectivity of so-called "randomized and blind" video-ratings.

2. The severity of the movement disorder was assessed before and after treatment by the patients and by the investigators using a 0-4 point rating scale. Randomized videotapes were rated by an independent neurologist with the global scale and the TSUI-scale. Although we found a high correlation (r> 0.6) of all scales in our study, they only measure approximately and show great discrepancies in some patients. Other studies (3) showed differences between the favourable evaluation by the patients and a markedly worse assessment by the investigators. In contrast, LORENTZ et al. 1992 found that patient self assessment is a reliable way of measuring treatment outcome (4). The TSUI-scale offers the best differentiation and the highest inter-rater reliability. Unlike the common procedure, statistic processing of rating scale scores must consider the values as ordinal scaled variables and use nonparametric statistics.

3. In our study EMG guided injection was only occasionally needed in complex patterns of muscle involvement. EMG can show the decrease of activity of a definite muscle before and after treatment (2). However, EMG can not reflect the clinical change of a complex movement pattern. Other instrumental methods like sonographic assessment of the injected sternocleidomastoid muscle can quantify the atrophy, but can not describe a clinical change (5).

4. Applied psychological tests can elucidate the relation between the "mechanistic" correction of a movement disorder and the course of coincident psychosocial and psychopathological disturbances. Our results indicate, that pre-treatment abnormalities disappear after months and years of successfull long-term treatment.

5. In the long-term studies reported, many important parameters are not well defined: "duration of benefit" (in our study 14 weeks) leads to the misunderstanding, that there exists a clear cut between "still benefit" and "recurrence of symtoms". However, waning benefit after the therapeutic peak effect is a continuous course and the patient expresses a need for reinjection according to his subjective perception. Patients impression that symptoms recur may be different from the investigators assessment.

There is no doubt, that injection of Botulinum toxin A is a simple and effective treatment of cervical dystonia. However one should face the fact, that unsolved methodical problems still exist and affect the evelution of the therapeutic efficacy as well as the comparability of different studies.

References:

1. Burke RE, Fahn S, Marsden CD, Bressmann SB, Moskowitz C, Friedman J (1985) Validity and reliability of a rating scale for the primary torsion dystonias. Neurology 35: 73-77.
2. Deuschl G, Heinen F, Kleedorfer B, Lücking CH, Poewe W (1992) Clinical and polymyographic investigation of spasmodic torticollis. J Neurol 239: 9-15.
3. Gelb DJ, Lowenstein DH, Aminoff MJ (1989) Controlled trial of botulinum toxin injections in the treatment of spasmodic torticollis. Neurology 39: 80-84.
4. Lorentz I, Davies L (1992) Validation of patient self assessment in botulinum treatment of spasmodic torticollis. Movement Disorders 7, Suppl 1: 136.
5. Schelosky L, Bergh B, Zendel W, Wissel J, Ebersbach G, Poewe W (1992) Sonographical assessment of sternocleidoid muscles in cervical dystonia pre and post botulinum toxin treatment. Movement Disorders 7, Suppl. 1: 132.

11

Scalp Potentials Preceeding Self Initiated Saccades to Visual Targets

W. Klostermann, D. Kömpf, R. Verleger, W. Heide,
B. Wauschkuhn, T. Seyfert
Neurologische Klinik, Medizinische Universität zu Lübeck

Similar to the readiness potential observed prior to limb movements, a presaccadic negativity (PSN) prior to saccades can be observed. We studied the PSN preceding voluntary, self-initiated saccades under two conditions:
1. saccades to a fixed visual target in the right hemifield,
2. saccades to the remembered target position in total darkness.
Methods: 10 right-handed students made saccades of 6° from a spot in the center to a second spot on the right side. EEG was recorded at 19 electrodes placed according to the international 10-20-system with a time constant of 5 sec.. A presaccadic interval of 8 sec. was averaged, triggered by the saccade onset in the horizontal EOG. Epochs with artifacts in the last 4 sec. prior to the saccades were excluded. The baseline was corrected referred to the average value over the interval [-4000 msec. | -3500 msec.] prior to saccade onset. To avoid the influence of accidental EEG background activity, the mean value of 80 msec.-intervals was used for statistics (paired t-test) and for amplitude mapping.
Results: The grand average of 10 subjects showed PSN onset 3 s prior to the saccades and maximum amplitude at the vertex (8 μV), equally for both conditions. A statistically significant difference of the PSN from baseline was seen at 13 electrodes in the "visual condition" and at 9 electrodes in the "remembered condition". Before PSN onset there was an isoelectrical plateau of 2 s duration, indicating that artifacts - caused by the preceding saccades - had returned to baseline. The PSN was more prominent over the (left) hemisphere contralateral to the saccade direction than over the ipsilateral hemisphere. Statistically significant differences were P3 > P4 (p< 0.01), C3 > C4, T3 > T4, T5 > T6 (p< 0.05) in the "visual condition" and F7 > F8, F3 > F4, T3 > T4 (p< 0.05) in the "remembered condition". A marked PSN over the parietal cortex was only present in the "visual condition" over the left hemisphere. In contrast, in the "remembered condition" there was a more pronounced PSN over the frontal cortex. Before saccades to the visual target there was a transitory, circumscribed maximum at an electrode placed between F3 and C3 ("FC3").
Conclusions: In our study, subjects performed intentional saccades that were visually guided in the first condition and memory guided in the second condition. In both conditions PSN onset and maximum were the same. The PSN maximum at the vertex is the same as seen prior to limb movements. It is supposed to reflect activity of the supplementary motor area, in our case especially the supplementary eye field. The marked PSN over the left parietal cortex in the "visual condition" might be attributed to directed visual attention to the right, contralateral hemifield, where the saccade target was located. The observation of a more pronounced PSN over the frontal cortex in the "remembered condition" fits to the results of studies in patients and to lesion experiments in monkeys, which show that frontal lobe lesions impair non-visually guided intentional saccades. Conversely, parieto-occipital lesions impair visually guided intentional saccades. A transitory, circumscribed maximum at the FC3-electrode prior to saccades to a visual target might reflect the activity of the contralateral frontal eye field.

12

SACCADIC DEFICITS IN UNILATERAL FRONTAL LOBE LESIONS

C. Mierisch, W. Heide, A. Moser and D. Kömpf
Dept. of Neurology, Medical University, Ratzeburger Allee 160, DW-2400 Lübeck, GERMANY.

Saccadic disorders after chronic unilateral cortical lesions are usually not obvious for the clinician and can only be diagnosed in a special behavioural context of the experimental paradigm. Using infrared reflection oculography, we recorded different types of volitional and reflexive saccades in 15 patients with unilateral lesions of the dorsolateral or dorsomedial frontal lobes, due to vascular accidents (7 cases) or tumour surgery (8 cases), 0.5 to 21 months (mean 6.6) prior to examination. Lesions predominantly involved the frontal eye fields (FEF) in 7 cases (4 right and 3 left hemispheric), the dorsolateral prefrontal cortex (Brodmann's area 46) in 4 cases (1 right and 3 left hemispheric) and the left supplementary motor area (SMA) in 3 cases. One patient had a subcortical lesion of the right fronto-temporal white matter, this was the only case with contralateral optic ataxia of visually elicited hand movements. Results were compared to an age-matched normal control group (n=30).
The saccadic main sequences of all patients were within normal limits, and visually guided saccades had normal latencies and amplitudes. Like in normal subjects, express saccades (with latencies of less than 150 msec) could be suppressed in the overlap paradigm (simultaneous presentation of the peripheral target and the fixation point); but in the gap paradigm (gap of 200 msec between extinction of the fixation point and onset of the peripheral target), the rate of express saccades was significantly reduced in patients with right FEF lesions, more pronounced into the contralateral hemifield. In antisaccade and remembered saccade tasks, however, most patients had deficits in suppressing inappropriate reflexive saccades, with an error rate of 30% to 80%, particularly if lesions included the frontal eye fields. Furthermore, the initiation of voluntary saccades (predictive, memory-guided or anti-saccades) was impaired in most patients with FEF or SMA lesions, in terms of increased latencies, whereas their amplitudes were within normal limits (except the case with optic ataxia, who showed low-gain memory-guided saccades into the contralateral hemifield).
In visual exploration tasks, only patients with right FEF lesions or bigger leisons of the left FEF) showed a preference for the ipsilateral hemifield. This contralateral visual exploration deficit was stimulus dependent, being more obvious when subjects had to scan an abstract visual scene (coloured squares) than when looking at a meaningful picture or when searching a letter. Furthermore, the frequency of exploratory saccades was diminished in those cases. None of these subjects had manifest visual hemineglect, but some of them showed a slight ipsilateral preference of spontaneous saccades in the dark, associated with minor deficits of spatial orientation or contralateral visual attention in adequate neuropsychological tests.
In conclusion, our results support the idea that the frontal lobes, particularly the frontal eye fields, play a major role in the cortical control of volitional saccades as well as in the volitional suppression of reflexive saccades, with a dominant influence on saccades into the contralateral hemifield.

13

PROCESSING OF VISUAL PATTERNS IN PATIENTS WITH UNILATERAL BRAINLESIONS: AN ANALYSIS WITH EVENT RELATED POTENTIALS

M. Matzke[1], H.J. Heinze[1], G. Dorfmüller[2], T.F. Münte[1], H. Dietz[2]
[1]Neurologische Klinik mit Klinischer Neurophysiologie
[2]Neurochirurgische Klinik der Medizinischen Hochschule Hannover

Recent studies have suggested that the posterior temporal cortex plays an important role in the perception of visual patterns. For example, in primates with lesions in the area of the superior temporal gyrus, deficits of visual discriminative functions were found. This has been corroborated in studies with humans. The present study aimed to the validate and extend those results by means of event-related brain potentials (ERP) and sought to pinpoint the neuronal mechanisms involved.

ERPs can be recorded non-invasively from the scalp and have been shown to vary systematically as a function of cognitive processing. Unlike behavioral measures they permit an on-line analysis of successive stages of information processing as several components have been associated with specific processing stages.

To investigate the question of whether there are hemispheric differences in the processing of visual patterns, we studied patients with unilateral lesions (CVA, slowly growing tumors) in the left (N=8) and right (N=10) temporo-parietal area as well as a control group (N=18). All patients were right-handed, had no visual-field deficits and had normal or corrected-to-normal vision. On a video monitor hierarchical letter stimuli were presented that were made up from larger letters (global level) formed by smaller letters (local level). For example, there would appear a large "H" made up of small "A"s. The subjects had to detect an assigned target letter regardless of the level at which it appeared. During the execution of the task we recorded behavioral- and ERP-measures that were analysed seperately for the global and local level. ERPs were recorded from 10 electrodes from standard left- and right-hemisphere scalp sites. They were averaged after using an automatic artifact-rejection system. The analysis yielded an enhanced negativity (N250) to the target letters in the 200-400 ms range poststimulus. This component was largest over the posterior temporal scalp sites and represented the earliest sign of a differential global/local target processing.

When the data of left-hemisphere damaged patients were analysed, a reduced N250 amplitude was found for the target letters at the global level. In contrast, the right-hemisphere damaged patients exhibited an inverted pattern of results with a reduction of N250 amplitudes for target letters on the local level. The analysis of the error rate similarily implicated an impairment for processing of global stimuli in the right-hemisphere and difficulties in local perception for the left-hemisphere patients, whereas the reaction times did not show any significant difference.

Thus, ERPs strongly support the notion of seperate processing of the global composition as opposed to local features of hierarchical stimuli. Our lesion study furthermore supports the view of a functional asymmetry of the hemispheres in the processing of visual hierarchical stimuli. Different levels of visual processing seemed to be impaired in patients with left as compared to right lesions of the temporo-parietal cortex. The N250 modulation in the lesion-group suggests that an early perceptual level of visual processing is impaired in the patients.

To summarize, these results provide further evidence for the important role of the temporo-parietal cortex in the analysis of hierarchical visual stimuli. Hemispheric differences in the perception of global and local information could be delineated. The ERP method significantly augments the previous results obtained in reaction-time studies.

14

Suppression of the visual perception by magnetic stimulation of the brain is delayed in patients with neuritis of the optic nerve

Masur, H., Papke, K., Oberwittler, C.
Department of Neurology, University of Münster, FRG

It was the purpose of the study to evaluate the clinical usefulness of the suppression of visual perception by magnetic stimulation [1] of the visual cortex in patients with optic neuritis.

Therefore, the influence of non-invasive stimulation of the brain on visual perception was examined in 15 patients with neuritis of the optic nerve. In all our cases the neuritis of the optic nerve was due to certain or probable encephalomyelitis disseminata. Only patients with typical clinical symptoms and delayed visual evoked potentials (VEP) were included.

3 letters were presented with a tachistoscope for 1 ms (white letters on a black ground). Letters were 4 mm high. The distance between the stimuli and the eyes was 50 cm. The visual perception was dependant on the brightness of the surrounding and the contrast on the screen. The magnetic stimulation was performed with an intensity of 1.5 tesla placing the coil over the occipital cortex. The time intervall between presentation of the visual stimulus and the application of the magnetic stimulus could be freely determined.

The results of our patients were compared with the data obtained in 20 age matched healthy individuals. Additionally, we correlated the latency of the maximal visual suppression with the latency of the visually evoked P 100.

The 15 patients showed different pathological conditions: (1) Complete inability to read the letters even if presented for an indefinite duration without subsequent magnetic stimulation (2 eyes), (2) inability to recognize the letters if they are presented tachistoscopically without subsequent transcranial stimulation (4 eyes), (3) lack of a clearcut suppression interval because of high background failure to report the letters correctly after subsequent transcranial stimulation (3 eyes), or (4) a clearcut suppression of visual perception after noninvasive stimulation of the visual cortex (21 eyes).

The mean latency of the maximal visual suppression was 105.7 ms +/- 16.5 ms (standard deviation) in patients with neuritis of the optic nerve and 80.75 ms +/- 11.2 ms (SD) in healthy volunteers. The comparison between the two groups revealed a significant difference (p < 0.01). The correlation between the latency of the maximal visual suppression and the latency of the P 100 (VEP) was r = 0.74.

In patients with neuritis of the optic nerve (prolonged VEP) the time intervall of reduced perception was delayed and prolonged. These findings agree very well with the hypothesis that the neuritis of the optic nerve produces a delay and a desynchronisation of the nerve action potentials. It may be presumed that the delay results in a shift of the suppression to higher latencies whereas the desynchronisation causes an increased width of the suppression interval. This methode provides the possibility to separate patients with neuritis of the optic nerve from normal individuals and to examine different perceptual functions.

1. Amassian VE, Cracco RQ, Maccabee PJ, Cracco JB, Rudell A, Eberle L (1989) Suppression of visual perception by magnetic coil stimulation of human occipital cortex. Electroenceph Clin Neurophysiol 74: 458-462

15

Pathogenesis of Vascular Ocular Syndromes

Müller M, Kessler Ch, Wessel K, [1]Mehdorn E, Kömpf D
Departments of Neurology and [1]Ophthalmology,
Medizinische Universität zu Lübeck, Lübeck, F.R.G.

We prospectively investigated 83 consecutive patients with vascular ocular syndromes. Nineteen patients had amaurosis fugax attacks (one bilaterally), 23 patients had occlusions of the central retinal artery or a branch retinal artery occlusion, 26 patients had a central retinal vein occlusion or a branch retinal vein occlusion (two bilaterally), and another 15 had anterior ischemic optic neuropathy (two bilaterally). 5 patients had bilateral symptoms, thus a total of 88 eyes were affected. All patients underwent a neurological examination, an examination of the visual evoked potentials as well as ultrasound investigations of the carotid arteries including continuous wave-Doppler sonography and duplex ultrasound.

Stenosis of more than 50% diameter reduction and occlusion of the internal carotid artery ipsilateral to the symptomatic eye were significantly more frequent in amaurosis fugax attacks (9/20) and central or branch retinal artery occlusion (7/23) than in central or branch retinal vein occlusion (1/28) or anterior ischemic optic neuropathy (0/17; $p \leq$ 0.025). Additionally, the analysis of plaque surface and echogenicity of the plaques on the affected side with a high resolution duplex scan uncovered that ulcerated plaque surfaces and plaques with a heterogeneous echogenicity were found significantly more frequent in the internal carotid arteries of patients with amaurosis fugax attacks (ulcerated 10/14, heterogeneous 11/16) and central or branch retinal artery occlusions (ulcerated 7/11; heterogeneous 9/14) than in patients with anterior ischemic optic neuropathy (ulcerated 0/6; heterogeneous 1/6; p< 0.05) or central and branch retinal vein occlusion (ulcerated 3/15; heterogeneous 3/17; $p \leq$ 0.025). Visual evoked potentials were significantly more delayed in patients with anterior ischemic optic neuropathy (4/8) as compared to patients with amaurosis fugax attacks (1/15) and central or branch retinal artery occlusion (1/17; p< 0.05). We conclude that amaurosis fugax attacks and central retinal artery or branch retinal artery occlusions are due to arterio-arterial embolization from ulcerated and heterogeneous carotid artery plaques, whereas anterior ischemic optic neuropathy is a disease of the small vessels affecting the posterior ciliary arteries with demyelinisation of the optic nerve.

16

Prognosis of visual acuity in eyes with vitreous hemorrhages due to an acute intracranial bleeding (Terson's Syndrom).

K.A. Baez [1], G. Hamann [2], H. Höh [1], K.W. Ruprecht [1]

[1] University Eye Hospital and Department, W-6650 Homburg (Saar), Germany
[2] University Neurology Department, W-6650 Homburg (Saar), Germany

Terson was the first to describe the oculo-cerebral syndrome in 1900 which associates intravitreal and retinal hemorrhages with subarachnoid bleedings. They are found in 20-40% of patients suffering from subarachnoid bleedings. Ocular hemorrhages are probably caused by a sudden increase of intracranial pressure which leads to a rupture of epi- and peripapillary capillaris due to consecutive increased intraocular pressure. Twelve eyes of ten patients with intraocular hemorrhages and intracerebral bleedings were enrolled in this study. All cases were treated in a neurological ICU and underwent secundary neurosurgical intervention. Mean age was 48 year (range 36-67). Visual acuity ranged from hand motions to 20/200 at the time of neurosurgery. In seven eyes a spontaneus resorption of intraocular blood was found within six months. Visual acuity in these eyes recovered to mean 20/25 (range 20/60 - 20/20) after two years. In the remaining five eyes a pars-plana vitrectomy was performed after 4 to 12 months following trauma. Visual acuity recovered to mean 20/25 (range 20/200 - 20/20) after two years. All eyes showed increased visual acuity following spontaneous resorption of intraocular blood or surgically removed hemorrhages. Reduced postoperative visual acuity was due to the development of a retinal detachment in two eyes and cataracts in three eyes.

Conclusion: In eyes with intraocular hemorrhage associated with acute intracranial subarachnoid hemorrhages (Terson's Syndrome) satisfying anatomical and functional results are gained by pars-plana vitrectomy if there is lack of spontaneous resorption of intraocular blood.

References:

1. Schultz PN, Sobol WM, Weingeist TA: Long-term-visual outcome in Terson's Syndrome. Ophthalmology, 98: 1814-19, 1991.

2. Broderick JP, Brott T, Tomsick T, et al.: The risk of subarachnoid and intracerebral hemorrhages in blacks as compared with whites. New Engl. J. Med. 326: 733-36, 1992.

3. Weingeist TA, Goldmann EJ, Folk JC, et al.: Terson's Syndrom. Clinicopathologic Correlations. Ophthalmology 93:1435-42, 1986.

4. Werry H, Brewitt H: Pars-plana Vitrektomie beim Terson-Syndrom. Fortschr. Ophthalmolol. 79: 424-27, 1983

17

INTRAARTERIAL FIBRINOLYSIS IN OCCLUSION OF THE CENTRAL RETINAL ARTERY

M. Schumacher, D. Schmidt, A.K. Wakhloo

Purpose: Acute central retina artery occlusion (CRAO) treated by any known conservative procedure has a poor prognosis. The study introduces intraarterial thrombolysis as a new treatment in CRAO which is expected to have better results than conservative methods.

Methods: We have treated 17 patients with intraarterial fibrinolysis, a method already in use for thrombo-embolic occlusion of the cerebral arteries. Fibrinolysis was carried out through a microcatheter placed supraselectively within the origin of the ophthalmic artery. In most cases urokinase was used in doses of between 200,000 and 1 Million units (in 5 patients rTPA was used instead).

Results: Five patients showed marked improvement or total recovery, and six more partial recovery, with improvement of the visual acuity or a field defect. The worst results were observed in the six patients where the mean delay between the appearance of clinical symptoms and initiation of treatment was more than 20 hours.

Discussion: Intraarterial thrombolysis has led to a better outcome in acute occlusion of the central retinal artery compared with conservative treatment. In those cases in which the ophthalmic artery cannot be supraselectively catheterized, treatment can be administered indirectly via the maxillary- ophthalmic collaterals. Analysis of the results shows that a good prognosis is to be expected when treatment starts within the first 6-8 hours, when there is some remaining visual function and less retinal edema.

References

1. Brückner R. Netzhautarterienverschluß. Der informierte Arzt - Gazette Médicale 1990; 6: 489-493

2. Schumacher M, Schmidt D, Wakhloo AK. Intraarterielle Fibrinolyse bei Zentralarterienverschluß. Radiologe 1991; 240-243

3. Karjalainen K. Occlusion of central retinal artery and retinal branch arterioles. A clinical, tonographic and fluorescein angiographic study of 175 patients. Acta Ophthalmol. Suppl. 1971; 109: 9-96

4. Augsburger JJ, Margal LE. Visual prognosis following treatment of acute central retinal artery obstruction. Br. J. Ophthalmol. 1980; 64: 913 - 917

18

Influence of visual stimuli on the dynamics of reactive perfusion changes in the posterior cerebral artery territory

I. Wittich, J. Klingelhöfer, G. Matzander, B. Conrad

Department of Neurology, Technical University of Munich, Möhlstraße 28, W-8000 München 80

Transcranial Doppler ultrasonography allows continuous on-line recordings of flow velocity changes corresponding to rapid alterations of the functional state. It was the aim of the present study to investigate qualitatively and quantitatively the influence of defined visual stimuli on the dynamics of flow velocity reactions in the posterior cerebral artery territory.

Recordings were made simultaneously from the posterior cerebral artery (P2-segment) in 16 right-handed healthy subjects using pulsed Doppler systems (2 MHz) unilaterally or bilaterally simultaneously while the subjects were regarding complex pictures 1) in the form of a half-field presentation, 2) into three viewing angles correlated with the 0.5, 0.2 and 0.04 isopters of the eye, 3) in presentation times of 50, 100 and 150 ms, 4) with and without searching task. Coloured slides were projected onto a screen (mean maximum illumination density 61 cd/m^2, viewing angle of 90° horizontally and 67.4° vertically, isopters-correlated viewing angle of 4.4/20.0/86.6° horizontally and 3.0/14.0/61.4° vertically). The first two stimulation tasks were presented while the subjects were fixating on a small red laser dot in the center of the screen.

In the simultaneous recording of the P2-segments during half-field stimulation, a significant ($p < 0.001$) increase in contralateral flow velocity could be observed (ipsilateral 10.04 % ± 7.76 %, contralateral 29.87 % ± 10.71 %). The flow velocity increase in the right posterior cerebral artery in both contralateral and ipsilateral half-field stimulation was significantly ($p < 0.001$) higher than on the left side. In full-field stimulation, this asymmetry was found to be less pronounced but still significant ($p < 0.01$). Viewing angle and flow velocity increase showed a positive correlation. Using brief presentation times, the onset of the reactive velocity increase clearly lagged behind the stimulus offset. In most cases presentation times of as little as 50 ms resulted in an increase of the perfusion. Blood flow velocity increase was steeper and attained higher values for the searching mode, when compared to the viewing mode for a given picture.

The significantly higher flow velocity increases during half-field and full-field stimulation in the right posterior cerebral artery are possibly attributable to different hemisphere-specific brain functions in right-handed subjects. In transition from small to medium and medium to large viewing angle flow velocity increased by the factors 1.4 and 1.8 despite an increase of the stimulus area by the factors 22 and 553 respectively. This can be attributed to the retinal receptor density which is substantially lower in the periphery and the associated disproportionately higher representation of retinal central fields in the visual cortex. Visual stimuli of different retinal extent and location on the one hand and the mode of stimulus perception on the other hand caused function-related flow velocity changes in defined cortical areas participating in visual information processing.

19

FUNCTIONAL CORTICAL INTERACTION PATTERNS IN VISUAL PERCEPTION AND VISUOSPATIAL PROBLEM SOLVING

H.L. Lagrèze, A. Hartmann, G. Anzinger
Neurologische Universitätsklinik, Bonn

Background: Large-scale neuronal networks subserving higher cortical functions in humans have been hypothesized on clinical and experimental grounds. Largely for methodological reasons functional neuro-imaging evidence is scarce. Multivariate analysis of regional cortical blood flow (rCBF) responses to behavioral activation may be a useful tool to study functional cortical interaction patterns in humans.

Methods: rCBF was measured by Xenon-133 clearance in 32 bihemispheric regions-of-interest in normal volunteers at rest, during a visual figures comparison task (n=35), and during a visuospatial problem solving task (n=39). Significant (p<0.01) interregional interactions were determined by partial correlation coefficients (removing global flow effects) between all regional flow increases, and factor analysis was used to describe the overall interregional covariance patterns.

Results: Significant rCBF increases ocurred in regions having specific subfunctions for each paradigm. Both tasks activated rCBF in bilateral premotor, motor, parietal and occipital regions. Bilateral prefrontal activation occurred during problem solving but not during the figures comparison task. Partial correlations coefficients and factor analysis identified significant inter-actions between numerous cortex regions in both tasks. There were highly ordered, non-random interaction patterns between these regions but also functional links to other cortex areas having non-significant flow increases.
Integrated patterns of functional interactions were seen between cortex areas subserving sub-functions of complex behavior. These statistical associations agreed with anatomic fiber connections known from experimental non-human primate studies.

Conclusions: Meaningful cortical interactions can be visualized by multivariate analysis of rCBF-responses to behavioral stimulation. Functional cortical networks are identified in the intact brain which enlarge the present neurophysiologic under-standing of higher brain functions. Cortical inter-action analysis by such techniques is a useful tool to describe the functional anatomy of large-scale neurocognitive networks in the intact human brain. Imaging functional interactions between active cortex areas is complementary to other experimental neurophysiologic methods to explore brain-behavior relationships in health and disease.

20

PHENOMENOLOGY OF VISUAL AGNOSIAS: THE SIGNIFICANCE OF CENTRAL DISORDERS OF OCULOMOTOR SYSTEMS

J.-N. PETROVICI, K. NIKLAUS
Department of Neurology, Cologne-Merheim

By the term visual agnosia, which we retain despite criticisms leveled against it, one refers to disorders of visual recognition that cannot be explained by a general disturbance of mental functioning or by a defect of elementary visual sensory function alone.
In four patients presenting with visual agnosias (two cases of visual object agnosia and two cases of Balint's syndrome) oculomotor disorders without evidence of periphere alterations of eye move-ments were found, such as disturbances of the convergence, defec-tive fixation and gaze instability. In all cases bilateral lesions affecting the parietooccipital areas were demonstrated.
Electrooculographic studies have been used to investigate two features of oculomotor dysfunction: the wandering of gaze in the search for an object to fixate on and the rigidity of fixation once the object has been discovered. . The electrooculographic records during the following of contours of letters drawn in the air by the examiner showed very slow and ample deflexions, thus correspon-ding to the grasp of the gaze. Whenever the patient could not follow a moving target with his eyes or any slowly moving object sudden abrupt deflexions were recorded, corresponding to the wandering gaze in search of a significant cue. No large saccades necessary for relating different portions of a visual scene were found, visual scanning was defective. This pattern of alterations was particulary evident in patients with Balint's syndrome. It may be seen that although from the clinical standpoint the pattern of the fixity of the gaze prevailed, the electrooculographic records showed a wandering of the gaze, which is evidence of the fact that the two patterns are closely linked in varying degrees of intensity.
Our findings justify a renewed discussion about the role of central oculomotor disorders in the production of agnosic phenomena. Vision is not a passive process. Normal vision involves more than the progressive extraction of critical spatial and temporal features of an input. It involves an intentional, active motor system compo-nent. Because the lesions that produce visual agnosia are cortical, the above oculomotor defects, which accompany the disorders of visual recognition, are cortical processing defects. The importance of defective visual field and arousal in eliciting visual agnosias will have to be elucidated by further research. The term agnosia does not imply a single underlying neuropsychological process that, when damaged, leads to the different syndromes. Regardless of interpretation, the evidence from clinical behavioral observations, experimental studies in human beings and animals, and anatomo-clinical correlations justify the acceptance of the visual agnosias as a special group of perceptual defects. The presence of confusio-nal states or general intellectual impairment cannot be invoked to explain the high degree of specificity found for some disorders of visual recognition.

21

COMPARISON OF MRI MORPHOLOGY AND OCULOMOTOR FUNCTION IN IDIOPATHIC CEREBELLAR ATAXIA

J.B. Schulz, M. Fetter, T. Klockgether, J. Faiss[1], E. Koenig, J. Dichgans

Neurologische Klinik und Abteilung für Neuroradiologie[1], Universität Tübingen, Hoppe-Seyler-Str. 3, D-7400 Tübingen, Germany

We compared the results of extensive oculomotor testing with computer aided planimetric evaluation of infratentorial atrophy by magnetic resonance imaging (MRI) in 17 patients with idiopathic cerebellar ataxia (IDCA) and 15 age-matched controls [3]. On the basis of their clinical presentation, patients were subdivided in one group with a pure cerebellar syndrome (IDCA-C, n = 7) and another group with additional non-cerebellar symptoms (IDCA-P, n = 10). Since clinical presentation is always almost purely cerebellar at disease onset, patients with a history of less than 4 years were excluded from this study [1]. Patients with additional symptoms (IDCA-P) usually have olivo-ponto-cerebellar-atrophy, whereas those with a purely cerebellar syndrome have cortical cerebellar atrophy.

Compared to normals MRI measurements showed significant atrophy in both patient groups of the cerebellar flocculi, the cerebellar hemispheres, the anterior and dorsal vermis. Atrophic changes were most severe in the IDCA-P group. The amount of atrophy of the pontine tegmental region and the pons was significant for the IDCA-P group but not for the IDCA-C group. Furthermore, the IDCA-P patients showed a significant atrophy compared to the IDCA-C patients for these two structures.

The most severe oculomotor deficits could be mainly attributed to lesions involving the floccular region of the cerebellum [4] with disturbed smooth pursuit, optokinetic nystagmus (OKN), suppression of the vestibulo-ocular reflex (VOR) and gaze-evoked nystagmus. These symptoms correlated well with the amount of atrophy of the flocculus found in MRI. However, these correlations were not specific. The above mentioned oculomotor functions correlated equally well with the atrophy of the dorsal vermis and also in part of the pontine tegmental region, the pons and even of structures known not to be involved in eye movement generation such as anterior vermis and cerebellar hemispheres. This co-correlation of atrophy in a degenerative disease, which normally involves the whole cerebellum, is not surprising. There was no correlation between saccade velocity and the amount of brainstem atrophy indicating a relative sparing of saccadic burst neurons even in severe brainstem atrophy. In fact, a recent report [2] disclosed that all cases of spino-cerebellar degeneration with slow saccades were hereditary.

Although patients with additional extracerebellar deficits (IDCA-P) had more severe oculomotor deficits than patients with pure cerebellar ataxia without brainstem invovement (IDCA-C), the pattern of the oculomotor disturbances was not significantly different between the two groups. This lack of difference indicates that the main eye movement pathology in these patients evolves from cerebellar disease. Thus, while clinical examination, MRI and eye movement analysis may complement each other and add to the criteria that provide the correct diagnosis in patients with progressive ataxias, eye movement analysis alone is not sufficient to distinguish between patients with IDCA-C and IDCA-P.

References

[1] Klockgether T, Schroth G, Diener HC, Dichgans J (1990) Idiopathic cerebellar ataxia of late onset: natural history and MRI morphology. J. Neurol. Neurosurg. Psychiatry 53: 297-305

[2] Mizutani T, Satoh J, Morimatsu Y (1988) Neuropathological backround of oculomotor disturbances in olivopontocerebellar atrophy with special reference to slow saccade. Clin. Neuropath. 7: 53-61

[3] Wüllner U, Klockgether T, Petersen D, Naegele T, Dichgans J (1992) Magnetic resonance imaging (MRI) in hereditary and idiopathic ataxia. Neurology (in press)

[4] Zee DS, Yamazaki A, Butler PH, Gueger G (1981) Effects of ablation of the flocculus and paraflocculus on eye movements in primate. J. Neurophysiol. 46: 878-899

22

DEFICITS OF SACCADES AND VISUO-SPATIAL ORIENTATION DUE TO UNILATERAL POSTERIOR PARIETAL LESIONS

W. Heide, A. Moser and D. Kömpf
Dept. of Neurology, Medical University, Ratzeburger Allee 160, W-2400 Lübeck, GERMANY

Various clinical reports on patients with cerebral hemispheric lesions as well as experimental findings in primates have presented evidence that the posterior parietal lobe is important both for visuo-spatial orientation and for various types of eye movements, including the spatial and temporal programming of saccades to visual targets. In the present study, we investigated how deficits of these functions correlate to each other in 15 cases of unilateral posterior parietal lesions. As saccadic deficits in those cases are often not obvious to the clinician, we applied stimuli in a specific behavioural context, appropriate for the investigation of cortical function. Spontaneous, reflexive and intentional visually guided saccades as well as exploratory, memory-guided and anti-saccades were recorded using infrared reflection oculography. Furthermore, visual attention and visuo-spatial orientation were examined by application of simple neuropsychological tests, such as line bisection and shape cancellation tasks, copying figures, spontaneous drawing, completion of a geographical map, mental rotation and Money's road map test. For the assessment of the subjective straight ahead and the subjective visual vertical, subjects had to adjust a laser target or a line of light-emitting diodes, respectively, both in darkness and with optokinetic stimulation around the vertical or the roll axis, respectively. As control, we examined 30 age-matched normal adults.

Lesions were caused by cerebral ischemia in 13 cases and by tumour surgery in 2 cases, having occurred 0.5 to 21 (mean 7.6) months (in 1 case 72 months) prior to examination. Only one of these cases had a left hemispheric lesion, 9 had lesions restricted to the right posterior parietal cortex, always including the intraparietal sulcus and the adjacent upper part of the angular gyrus (Brodmann's area 39), and 6 had larger right parietal lesions extending into the temporal lobe. None of the patients had manifest visual field defects, 2 of them had hemiparesis. Eight patients (1 left and 7 right hemispheric) had mild or moderate optic ataxia, most pronounced for targets in the contralateral hemifield.

Manifest visual hemineglect was obvious at the time of examination in 3 right parietal cases, all with larger lesions extending into the central or temporal cortex. Six other patients (right parietal lesions) showed signs of impaired visual attention for the contralateral hemifield, either in the neuropsychological tests or - as an even more sensitive parameter - in terms of a contralateral deficit of exploratory eye movements, mostly associated with increased latencies and reduced amplitudes of visually guided saccades, more for contralateral than for ipsilateral saccades. The increase of saccadic latencies was significant (p<0.001) for the whole group of parietal patients, it was most pronounced when the fixation point remained on during presentation of the peripheral target (overlap paradigm), indicating that those parietal patients had problems to disengage visual attention from the present target. But even with extinction of the fixation point 200 msec prior to target onset, the percentage of short-latency express saccades (with latencies of less than 150 msec) was reduced in most parietal patients, as compared to normal adults. Voluntary saccades to remembered target locations or antisaccades also showed increased latencies in some of the patients, but the effect was weaker than for visually guided reflexive saccades. During those tasks, about half of the patients had deficits in suppressing inappropriate reflexive saccades, particularly in the antisaccade paradigm, but to a much lesser extent than patients with frontal lobe lesions. An ipsilateral shift of the subjective straight ahead, a contralateral tilt of the subjective visual vertical or an impaired perception of circular vection during optokinetic stimulation, particularly with contralateral half-field stimulation, were found in about 50% of the cases, but without a clear correlation with other visuo-spatial or ocular motor deficits or with the presence of optic ataxia.

In conclusion, exploratory and visually guided saccades are a sensitive indicators for subclinical deficits of visual attention, in good accordance with neuropsychological findings. Furthermore, the posterior parietal cortex is particularly important for the spatio-temporal control of visually guided reflexive saccades. To a minor extent, it seems to be involved also in the initiation of voluntary saccades, which is more a function of frontal areas, like the voluntary suppression of reflexive saccades. Visuo-motor coordination of goal-directed arm movements, visually elicited self-motion sensation and the maintainance of a stable internal representation of visuo-spatial coordinates seem to be mediated by different parts of the posterior parietal cortex, because there was no clear correlation between these functions and saccadic performance in most parietal patients.

23

Visual Extinction Demonstrated With The Scanning Laser Ophthalmoscope

A. Rosengart[1], R.F. Kaplan[2], T.R. Hedges III.[3], A.E. Elsner[4], L.R. Caplan[2]

Klinik für Neurologie[1], Medizinische Universität zu Lübeck, Lübeck, FRG; Department of Neurology[2] and Neuro-ophthalmology[3], New England Medical Center and Eye Research Institute[4], Boston, USA

Extinction to double simultaneous stimulation (DSS) refers to a failure to detect 1 of 2 simultaneously presented stimuli, even though when presented individually each stimulus can be detected successfully. The present report describes preliminary data from an ongoing study of the spatial and temporal parameters of extinction in right hemisphere damaged (RHD) patients using the laser scanning ophthalmoscope (SLO). The SLO enables the time controlled presentation of stimuli to specific locations of the retina. The objectives of this study are: (I.) to demonstrate the attentional deficits in clinically normal RHD patients; (II.) to exame the spatial and temporal parameters of retinal stimulation underlying the deficit; (III.) to further exame the effect of implicit cuing in shifting attention without corresponding eye movements.

The subjects were 2 patients with right hemisphere stroke and 3 age-matched normal controls. Both patients, examined 7 month and 4 years after their stroke, had shown evidence of left hemispatial neglect immediately following their stroke but were clinically normal on tests of letter cancellation and extinction to double simultaneous finger stimulation at the time of this study. A computer-controlled SLO provided a high quality video image of the retina and the generated stimuli. The timing was controlled by a Lafayette elctronic tachistoscope attachment. A retinal field of 29 x 23 degrees was illuminated by a light of 830nm. Light stimuli of 633nm at .1microW/cm^3 forming the letter "A" were 1.22 degrees high and 1.22 degrees wide. The difference of brightness between sti-muli and background was 1.92 log units. During 20 DSS trials, the 2 stimuli were 11.26 degrees apart and one was directed to either side of the fovea. DSS trials were preceded by 3 unilateral stimulation trials directed to either side of the fovea. An equal number of DSS trials were preceded by 3 right unilateral trials, 3 left uni-lateral trials, a single left unilateral trial, a single right unilateral trial and a single left unilateral trial. The stimuli were presented at 50, 100, or 200 msec.

Neither of the two controls showed extinction to DSS when the stimuli were presented at 50 msec, whereas both patients extingui-shed left-sided stimuli. Patient 1, a 38 year odl man with a right frontal lesion, correctly identified the location of all the unilateral stimuli but extinguished 1 of the 2 stimuli during 17.5% (5 left, 2 right) of the DSS trial at 50 msec. Patient 2, a 54 year old man with a large right fronto-parietal lesion, correctly identified unilaterally presented stimuli but extinguished the left-sided stimuli on every trial at 50 msec. At 100 msec, Patient 2 extinguished 1 of 2 stimuli only 25% of the DSS trials (8 left, 2 right). At 200 msec, Patient 2 performed perfectly on all DSS trials. The pattern of unilateral stimulation preceding a DSS trials did not appear to effect the probability of extinction for either patient. Neither of the 2 controls showed extinction to DSS when the stimuli were presented at 50 msec, whereas both patients extinguished left-sided stimuli. Patient 1, a 38 year odl man with a right frontal lesion, correctly identified the location of all the unilateral stimuli but extinguished 1 of the 2 stimuli during 17.5% (5 left, 2 right) of the DSS trial at 50 msec. Patient 2, a 54 year old man with a large right fronto-parietal lesion, correctly identified unilaterally presented stimuli but extinguished the left-sided stimuli on every trial at 50 msec. At 100 msec, Patient 2 extinguished 1 of 2 stimuli only 25% of the DSS trials (8 left, 2 right). At 200 msec, Patient 2 performed perfectly on all DSS trials. The pattern of unilateral stimulation preceding a DSS trials did not appear to effect the probability of extinction for either patient.

These data demonstrate that deficits of attention for visual space *persist following* recovery from the neglect syndrome. The phenomena of extinction during DSS is a function of temporal as well as the spatial constrains. Although both RHD patients showed a greater propensity for extinction of the left-sided stimulus, both also extinguished the stimulus on the right. Surprisingly, the probability of extinction was not effected by the preceding unilateral stimulus. We speculate that the role of small eye move-ments may be an important factor in shifting attention in neglect, although the focus of the lesion (frontal vs. parietal) may also to be prove to be a factor.

24

QUANTIFICATION OF OCULAR MISALIGNMENT IN NEURO-OPHTHALMOLOGICAL PATIENTS WITH PHOTO-GRAPHIC PURKINJE REFLECTION PATTERN EVALUATION

J.C. Barry[1], R. Effert[1], A. Kaupp[2]

[1]Eye Clinic, Head: Prof. M. Reim, Faculty of Medecine, RWTH University Aachen, Pauwelsstraße 30, D-5100 Aachen

[2]Lehrstuhl für Meßtechnik, Head: Prof. D. Meyer-Ebrecht, Faculty of Electric Engineering, RWTH University Aachen, Templergraben 55, D-5100 Aachen

A simple photographic method is presented to measure the exact amount of ocular misalignment under natural viewing conditions, at near or distance fixation, in primary, secondary and tertiary positions, with or without glasses.

As measuring principle, the **Purkinje Reflection Pattern Evaluation*** method is used: the relative positions of the anterior corneal reflection (1st Image of Purkinje) and the posterior reflection of the crystalline lens (4th Image of Purkinje) in the pupils can be used as parameters of gaze direction.

When using three horizontally aligned equidistant flashes three corneal reflections and three posterior lens reflections can be observed close to the pupil plane in each eye. These form a characteristic reflection pattern, consisting of two horizontal, parallel rows of smalls dots against the dark background of the pupil. The shift between the two rows of reflections it proportional to the angle between the optic axis of each eye and the symmetry axis of the flash set-up.

The recording of the two reflection patterns is done simultaneously with a 35mm reflex camera equipped with a 105mm macro-tele lens. The system is integrated in a chin/head rest examination stand. Specific gaze directions can be chosen with light emitting diodes used as fixation lights. For distance fixation, a tangent screen with light emitting diodes is used. Differentiation between paretic and concomitant strabismus can be done on comparing pictures taken in monocular and binocular fixation.

The evaluation of the photographically stored reflection patterns is done on the magnified slides by measuring the relative distances of the reflections and computing the angles of gaze position for each eye with a simple formula.

Advantages of this method are: simple, easy to use measuring principle; low cost; high accuracy of 1-3° depending on the measuring strategy; can be used if one eye cannot fixate; can be used in cases of nystagmus; simultaneous documentation of lid position and pupillary diameter with a built in mm-scale; exact reproduceability of gaze direction; orthoptically trained personel not necessary.

Selected cases of healthy subjects and patients are reported to illustrate the system´s performance for documentation, follow-up and differential diagnosis in neuro-ophthalmologic diseases, e.g. of supranuclear origin, with Reflection Pattern Evaluation.

*Barry JC, Effert R, Kaupp A (1992) Objective Measurement of Small Angles of Strabismus in Infants and Children with Photographic Purkinje Reflection Pattern Evaluation. Ophthalmology 99:320-328

25

Duane's Retraction Syndrome

Jerusalem, F., Z. Nüssgens, P. Roggenkämper
Bonn, Germany

Duane's syndrome is a sporadic or autosomal dominant disorder characterized by uni- or bilateral eyemuscle weakness with retraction of the eyeball and narrowing of the palpebral fissure.

Three types of Duane's retraction syndrome can be distinguished:
Duane I
Limitation or absence of abduction, normal or only slightly defective adduction, narrowing of the palpebral fissure and retraction of the affected eyeball on adduction, widening of the palpebral fissure on attempted abduction.
Duane II
Limitation or complete defect of adduction with exotropia of the affected eye. Abduction is normal or only slightly limited. Distinct narrowing of the palpebral fissure and retraction of the globe on attempted adduction.
Duane III
Limitation or absence of both abduction and adduction of the affected eye and retraction of the globe and narrowing of the palpebral fissure on attempted adduction.

Apart from the disorders of motility in the horizontal plane, frequently additional vertical motor anomalies can be observed. Electrophysiological and neuropathological findings suggest that Duane's syndrome is due to a developmental defective innervation of ocular muscles.

We observed 33 cases (10 adults, 23 children and adolescents; 22 females, 11 males). An unilateral defective ocular motility was observed in 21 cases (14 left, 7 right) and a bilateral defective ocular motility was observed in 12 cases. An abnormal head position was evident in 26 cases, this or cosmetic aspects were reasons for operative correction of defective ocular motility. 10 % of the patients complained about diplopia or headaches.

Duane's syndrome is an important consideration in the differential diagnosis of eye muscle weakness and can be readily diagnosed by simple inspection.

26

EYE MOVEMENT DISORDERS IN LATE ONSET CEREBELLAR ATAXIA

A. Wittkämper, W. Heide, K. Wessel, A. Moser and D. Kömpf
Dept. of Neurology, Medical University, Ratzeburger Allee 160, DW-2400 Lübeck, GERMANY

In 19 patients with hereditary or sporadic cerebellar ataxia of late onset, eye movements were recorded using DC-electrooculography. Computer-based data analysis was performed off-line, concerning saccadic, pursuit and optokinetic eye movements. According to clinical and neuroradiological criteria, 10 of these patients (group 3) were classified as olivo-ponto-cerebellar atrophies (OPCA) or multisystem atrophies, and 9 as pure cerebellar atrophies (CA), 3 of them (group 2) with abnormal electrophysiological findings (evoked potentials, blink reflex, long-loop reflexes), indicating subclinical brainstem or multisystem involvement.

All 19 patients showed oculomotor signs of cerebellar disease, such as low gain of smooth pursuit (89%) or optokinetic nystagmus (84%), impaired suppression of the vestibulo-ocular reflex (VOR) by visual fixation (100%) or head tilt (defective "dumping" of its time constant, like in lesions of the cerebellar nodulus and inferior vermis, 95%), saccadic dysmetria (84%, half of them with hypermetric saccades) and gaze-evoked nystagmus (47%), less frequently hyperexcitability of VOR (37%), square wave jerks with visual fixation (21%), increased saccadic latencies (21%) or rebound nystagmus (16%). Downbeat nystagmus was found in 2 cases (1 CA and 1 OPCA) and upbeat nystagmus in 1 case (pure CA). All these symptoms did not discriminate between CA and OPCA. Ocular motor signs of brainstem involvement, however, were present only in OPCA patients (80%), namely slow horizontal saccades (60%, all hereditary OPCA's), in 5 cases combined with upward vertical gaze palsy, or abnormally low VOR gain (<0.5 with sinusoidal or ramp stimuli of 90°/sec), mostly with time constants of less than 5 seconds (50%). Two manifest OPCA cases had purely cerebellar oculomotor symptoms, these were the only OPCA's with normal evoked potentials. On the other hand, the 3 CA patients with abnormal evoked potentials did not show any ocular motor signs of brainstem involvement. Statistical comparison of CA and OPCA cases revealed a significant reduction only of VOR gain in the OPCA group (p<0.05).

In conclusion, eye movement disorders are sensitive indicators of cerebellar ataxia. Particularly deficits of vestibulo-cerebellar functions (flocculus and nodulus) were present in all cases, such as incomplete fixation suppression of the VOR, defective head tilt dumping of the VOR time constant, low gain of smooth pursuit or optokinetic nystagmus. Furthermore, the ocular motor findings confirmed the clinical classification of OPCA and CA in most cases. Slow saccades, vertical gaze palsy and low VOR gain are specific OPCA symptoms, correlating with abnormal evoked potentials, although not present in all cases. The combination of slow saccades and vertical gaze palsy was found only in rapidly progressive, hereditary OPCA cases, indicating a special subgroup of the disease. For the electrophysiological signs of subclinical extracerebellar manifestation in 3 CA cases (group 2), we found no ocular motor correlate. In 3 pure CA cases of group 1, however, follow-up examinations must show, if the presence of upbeat nystagmus (1), increased saccadic latencies (3) or low-limit values for saccadic velocity or VOR gain (2) can predict the development of OPCA, as do abnormal evoked potentials.

27

Differential diagnosis of unexplained visual loss by means of the pupillary light reaction

H. Wilhelm, U. Schiefer, E. Zrenner
University Eye Hospital, Department of Pathophysiology of Vision and Neuro-ophthalmology, D-7400 Tübingen

Usually, both pupils are equal in diameter and react synchronously to light, even if the light sensitivity of one eye is severely reduced. In case of a unilateral disease there may be a difference in the pupillary light reaction evoked in both eyes, although the pupils still react synchronously. The light reaction obtained from the involved eye, however, is reduced in amplitude and velocity compared to that from the normal eye. Comparing the pupil light reaction elicited by repetitively directing the light first to one then to the other eye is an excellent method detecting an afferent pupillary defect. This test was introduced by Levatin in 1959 [2] and is known as the swinging flashlight test. It may be performed if the iris and its nervous input are unimpaired in both eyes. Therefore, before performing the swinging flashlight test, it has to made sure that there is no efferent pupillary defect, i.e. an anisocoria needs to be excluded at two different light levels and the pupils must of course both be able to react on light. If there is a defect in one eye (anisocoria, iris damage) it is still possible to detect an afferent pupillary defect by comparing the direct and indirect light reaction of the better reacting pupil. The most sensitive indicator of a minimal afferent defect is the initial pupillary constriction when the light is directed onto the eye [1]. In case of a more severe afferent defect the involved pupil will even dilate when the examination light returns from the normal eye. The best results are obtained with rather bright test light in a darkened examination room. To get reliable results the test has to be repeated several times. The difference between the examination time of involved and normal eye should be minimal, and the distance and angle with the optical axis must be the same in both eyes. An afferent defect can be simulated either by looking about 30 seconds into a strong light (e.g., ophthalmoscope) or, contralaterally, by patching one eye for half an hour. Those effects last only for about 5 minutes [5].

Afferent pupillary defects are only found in unilateral or asymmetrical diseases. In the latter case the expression "relative afferent pupillary defect" (RAPD) is preferred. Diseases of the optical media (refractive error, opacities) never cause RAPD, even if visual acuity is 20/20 in one eye and light perception in the other. A dense cataract with a RAPD indicates that there is something wrong with the function of the retina or the optic nerve [4,5]. The cause for the absence of RAPD in media opacities is probably a scattering of light directly onto the fovea enhanced by the increased amount of dark adaptation that results in a sensitivity increase. Retinal diseases only cause RAPD if they are very extensive and therefore ophthalmoscopically visible. Unilateral optic nerve diseases always cause RAPD. Therefore, the swinging flashlight test is an excellent method in differentiating an optic nerve disease from other causes of visual loss including feigned visual loss [4,5]. Chiasmal lesion can cause RAPD since they are often asymmetrical. Optic tract and lateral geniculate body lesions virtually always cause RAPD, retrogeniculate lesion only in one third. The cause for the RAPD in optic tract and part of retrogeniculate lesions is still unclear. Amblyopia may in some cases cause a small RAPD, independent from the degree of visual loss [3].

By means of neutral density filters the degree of RAPD may be measured quantitatively [5]. This method is very helpful if subjective measurements as visual acuity and visual fields fail.

The swinging flashlight test is an objective fast an easy method that offers valuable information about the cause and extent of visual loss. A normal swinging flashlight test excludes a unilateral optic nerve disease.

References:

1. Cox TA (1989) Pupillographic characteristics of simulated afferent pupillary defects. Invest Ophthalmol Vis Sci 30:1127-1131
2. Levatin P (1959) Pupillary escape in disease of the retina or optic nerve. Arch Ophthalmol 62:768-779
3. Portnoy JZ, Thompson HS, Lennarsson L, Corbett JJ (1983) Pupillary defects in amblyopia. Am J Ophthalmol 96:609-614
4. Thompson HS (1966) Relative afferent pupillary defects. Am J Ophthalmol 62:860-873
5. Wilhelm H (1991) Pupillenreaktionen — Pupillenstörungen. Kohlhammer Verlag, Stuttgart

28

Homonymous hemianopia due to cerebral infarction - The prognostic significance of phosphens

Hans W. Kölmel
(Department of Neurology, Humboldt University, Charité Berlin, Germany)

Introduction:
Phosphens are an expression of the discharge of visual neurons and result from stimuli located somewhere in the course of the visual pathway, most often in the retina, the lateral geniculate body or the occipital cortex. When they appear, one may assume that neuronal inhibition is deficient and that the structures responsible for generation and transmission of impulses are intact. They are relatively unspecific but become more useful as localizing signs when they appear as precursors or sequelae of defined neurological deficits. When they appear in a hemianopic field, then they are located in or near the lesion responsible for the visual field defect. In cases of cerebral ischemia, phosphens appearing in conjunction with homonymous hemianopia suggest that definitive destruction of neuronal structures has not occurred. Therefore, phosphens may be considered as evidence of potential recovery and as prognostically favourable signs.

Methods:
In order to determine the prognostic significance of phosphens in hemianopic fields, we studied 145 patients with brain infarction and homonymous visual field defects for periods ranging up to 6 years. For the purposes of the present study we limited our observations to 125 patients with clinical presentations and CT findings consistent with infarction in the distribution of the posterior cerebral artery. Patients were enroled if the clinical event had occurred within the preceding three weeks, and 85 % of patients were included within two days of the development of hemianopia. A semi-standardized questionnaire was used to elicit information on phosphens. On the basis of previous experience, we categorized phosphens as colourful, colouriess, bright or dull. Visual fields were measured with the Goldmann perimeter at regular intervals over a period of three months after the index event. Additional examinations were performed in patients who failed to recover during this period.

Results:
119 of 125 patients were evaluated. Phosphens were reported in 56 cases, and improvement in the visual field examination was recorded in 41 (73 %) of these patients. 63 patients did not experience phosphens, and improvement was documented in 34 cases (54 %). This represents a significantly better prognosis in the patients who experienced phosphens. Of 41 patients who experienced colourful phosphens fog was seen in 10 cases, fields in 9, and coloured patterns in 22 patients. 31 of these patients (75 %) improved (7 who saw fog, 7 with fields, and 17 with colourful patterns) - a significantly better result than in the group of patients without phosphens. The rate of improvement in the group of patients with colourful patterns was 77 %. Complete recovery from the visual field defect was observed most often in this group. 36 patients reported colourless phosphens and 26 (72 %) recovered.

Discussion:
The results demonstrate that patients with homonymous hemianopia following occipital infarction have a significantly better prognosis when phosphens appear in the affected visual field. The prognosis is especially favourable in cases with colourful patterns. These findings support the hypothesis that phosphens demonstrate the presence of a functioning neuronal network in the visual cortex.

References:
Gloning I, Gloning K, Hoff H (1967) Über optische Halluzinationen. Wien Z. Nervenheilkd 25: 1-19
Kölmel HW (1984) Visuelle Halluzinationen im hemianopen Feld. Schriftenreihe Neurologie Bd. 26, Springer, Berlin Heidelberg New York Tokyo

29

How Do Hemianopic Patients Read ?

Dieter Schoepf and W.H. Zangemeister
Neurological University Clinic Hamburg, FRG

Horizontal and vertical eye movements (DC-EOG) of normal subjects and ten patients with hemianopic visual field defects of different ätiology have been recorded for a basic quantification of their adaptive ocular motor and head strategies during reading. All subjects had to read aloud, most accurately, and time optimal, i.e quickly, four different short texts with distinct content: First in an experimental head fixed, second in a more natural head-free-to-move condition. Neglect phenomena was excluded in a complete neuropsychological testing.

The reading pattern of the normal subjects appeared to be stable, and it was in accordance with the classical `stop and go' reading pattern . This was accompanied by only few regressions, a short global reading time, and a synchronous horizontal torque and head movement pattern. Normal subjects were able to reduce their global reading time with forced head movements. Comparatively, only one of ten hemianopic patients was able to increase significantly his reading rate in the head-free-to-move condition. For both, normal readers and hemianopic patients, with forced head movements the number of positional fixation pauses was increased, whereas the number of lexical fixation pauses was decreased.

Hemianopic patients avoided larger head movements: Patients with left hemianopic visual field defects employed an adaptive side of attention change of head movements from the blind hemifield into the seeing hemifield with altogether reduced head movement amplitudes into both hemifields. Patients with right hemianopic visual field defects mostly used a `wait and see' head movement stategy with generally minimized head movements. They employed a consistent set of ocular motor reading strategies to compensate their visual handicap. Respectively, at the end of a line well adapted patients frequently used a `blind hemifield overshooting' strategy, whereas less adapted patients mostly used an ènd of line detective' strategy. Additionally, reading saccade amplitudes were reduced in size compared to normal readers. Hemianopic patients with left homonymous visual field defects demonstrated a `beginning of line detective' strategy with accumulation of saccades.

The reading rate of two patients which showed additional signs of visual hemiinattention during the neuropsychological tests was extremly decreased compared to the other hemianopic patients. The reading pattern appeared as `disorganized', and no kind of short adaptation was developed in ocular motor reading and head movement strategies.

30

OPTIC NERVE LESION IN CRANIOSYNOSTOSIS

H. Collmann(1), N. Sörensen(1).
J. Krauß(1), J. Sold(2), J. Mühling(3)

Dpt. Pediatric Neurosurgery(1), Opthalmology(2), Maxillo-facial Surgery(3), University Hospital, Würzburg

Deterioration of optic nerve function is the most serious consequence of severe longstanding craniostenosis. There are few comprehensive studies on the frequency and severity of optic nerve damage in various types of craniosynostosis.

During the last 10 years 496 patients treated for primary craniosynostosis at our institution were subjected to routine ocular examination prior to surgery. Fundoscopy was abnormal in 57 of them: Papilledema was noted in 29, and optic atrophy in the other 28 patients. Two out of 302 patients with isolated synostosis of a single suture had papilledema, none of them had optic atrophy. In contrast, from a total of 194 patients with multiple suture synostosis or with syndromous synostosis 28 percent suffered from some kind of optic nerve lesion. Patients with Crouzon's or Pfeiffer's disease were most frequently affected: 59 percent had signs of optic nerve lesion at fundoscopy. In 16 percent of them significant visual failure or even blindness was stated. Patients with Apert's or Chotzen's syndrome were at much less risk.

Only 39 percent of patients with intracranial hypertension due to craniostenosis presented with abnormal fundoscopic findings. Conversely, in several instances papilledema as well as optic atrophy turned out to be the only signs of craniostenosis, since clinical complaints were absent and radiological findings were inconclusive.

In all 28 patients presenting with optic atrophy at first examination intracranial hypertension could be substantiated. The history of 20 of them revealed some undue delay in diagnosis and surgical treatment of craniostenosis.

Conclusions:

1. Intracranial hypertension due to craniostenosis is the main if not single causative factor of optic nerve damage in craniosynostosis.

2. The risk to the optic nerve may be infered from the severity of the underlying craniosynostosis and the number of sutures fused.

3. The significance of optic nerve injury in syndromous craniosynostosis is still undererstimated.

4. Optic nerve injury may be overlooked since other signs of craniostenosis may be absent.

Poster session I
Ophthalmoneurology

31

Early and late suppression of the visual perception after non-invasive magnetic stimulation of the occiput

Papke, K., Masur, H., Oberwittler, C.

Department of Neurology, University of Münster, FRG

It was the aim of the investigation to study in detail different factors influencing the reduction or suppression of visual perception induced by non-invasive magnetic stimulation of the visual cortex. This method was first described by Amassian and colleagues in 1989 [1].

Therefore, the suppression of visual perception induced by non-invasive magnetic stimulation of the occipital area was examined in 20 healthy volunteers. 3 letters were presented as optic stimuli with a tachistoscope for 1 ms (white letters on a black ground). Letters were 4 mm tall on the screen. Subjects were placed 50 cm in front of a screen (20 x 30 cm) and presented slides showing a random set of 3 letters. The visual perception was dependant on the brightness of the surrounding and the contrast on the screen. Given the described experimental conditions, all healthy subjects were able to report the letters correctly, producing only occasional errors.

The magnetic stimulation was performed with an intensity of 1.5 tesla placing the coil (14 cm in diameter) tangentially over the occipital cortex. The time intervall between presentation of the visual stimulus and the application of the magnetic stimulus could be varied freely.

The suppression of visual perception was influenced by visual (brightness, contrast, duration) and by stimulus (intensity, coil placement) conditions.

The method showed a good intraindividual reproducibility. No significant differences between the usage of the right, left or both eyes were detected.

In 10 of 20 individuals a complete suppression could be obtained, in the 10 others only a partial suppression. In the first group (complete suppression) the maximum of the visual suppression was 73.5 ms with a standard deviation (SD) of 6.5 ms (for the le. eye) and 74.0 ms with a SD of 5.95 ms (for the ri. eye). In the second group (partial suppression) a maximal suppression of 94.2 ms +/- 10.7 ms (SD) (for the le. eye) and of 92.0 ms +/- 8.2 ms (SD) (for the ri. eye) was detected.

If the intensity of stimulation was reduced in individuals with a complete suppression a partial suppression could be observed with a latency corresponding to those of the second group. Partial suppression was always related to higher latencies of the maximal suppression.

The results indicate that the magnetic stimulation - dependant on the intensity of stimulation - interferes with the process of visual perception at different stages or sites of the visual pathways. Early complete suppression (requiring high stimulus intensity) points to a deep localization and the late incomplete suppression to a more superficial localization of the involved anatomical structure.

1. Amassian VE, Cracco RQ, Maccabee PJ, Cracco JB, Rudell A, Eberle L (1989) Suppression of visual perception by magnetic coil stimulation of human occipital cortex. Electroenceph Clin Neurophysiol 74: 458-462

32

OCCIPITAL P270 IN M.ALZHEIMER, RECORDED IN A VISUAL P300-PARADIGM
R. Verleger,
E. Wascher & D. Kömpf
Dept. of Neurology, Medical University at Lübeck

Frequently, event-related EEG potentials have been recorded from demented patients in tasks using auditory stimuli, but there are almost no reports about tasks in which visual stimuli were presented. Using such a visual task, we had found an occipital positive component, peaking at 270 msec, which component was markedly larger in Alzheimer patients than in healthy control subjects (Verleger et al. 1992). In that task, the words "push" and "wait" were presented in random order, with 50% probability each. In the auditory "oddball" task, however, that has been the usual paradigm in this area of research, the relevant stimulus (the "target") is presented much less frequently than in 50% of all stimuli. Therefore, in the present study we wanted to replicate this finding in a task that was more similar to the auditory "oddball" task.

Eight patients were studied, of which five had a dementia of the Alzheimer type, three of the vascular type. The degree of dementia was mild to moderate. In intervals of 1.5 sec, a large circle was flashed on a screen. The circle's color was blue in most cases (about 200 times) and sometimes yellow (about 50 times). Subjects had to press a button with the yellow circles. Recordings were made from Fz, Cz, Pz, Oz vs. linked mastoids, additionally from the eyes (above vs. below), with a time constant of 1 sec.

Both the vascular and the Alzheimer group of patients showed a large occipital positivity in the 250-300 msec interval following onset of the yellow circles. In age-matched control subjects, this component was markedly smaller.

Thus, the occipital P270 seems to be a regular phenomenon in dementia patients. It may be interpreted as the lack of a negativity in this time range, by this being similar to the often-replicated finding in the auditory oddball task where Alzheimer patients display a reduction of the N2b component. Both phenomena illustrate in high temporal resolution the interruption of information processing that takes place in the patients after they have regularly perceived the presented stimuli.

Reference: Verleger, R., Kömpf, D., & Neukäter, W. (1992) Event-related EEG potentials in mild dementia of the Alzheimer type. *Electroencephalography and Clinical Neurophysiology*, in press

33

Processing of visual information in dementia of Alzheimer type - correlation between positron emission tomography and fragmented picture test

R.Mielke, J.Kessler, G.R.Fink, K.Herholz, W.-D.Heiss

Max-Planck-Institut für Neurologische Forschung, Gleuelerstr.50, 5000 Köln 41, Germany

Objective and background. While neuropathological changes in dementia of Alzheimer type (DAT) are most pronounced in cortical association areas, primary sensory cortices are relatively unaffected. However, we have frequently noted DAT patients presenting with prominent basic and complex visual deficits. Consistent with the clinical heterogeneity these visual symptoms may attribute to either affection of extraocular motility, pregeniculate afferent pathways or cortical dysfunction (1). A subgroup of the latter is Balint's syndrome, in which spatial agnosia arises from dysfunction of visual association areas. Due to a close relationship between the regional cerebral metabolic rate of glucose (rCMRGl) and neuronal function positron emission tomography (PET) may elucidate alterations of functional networks involved in visual information processing in DAT subjects.

Methods and design. We studied 31 patients (mean age: 67.4 years, age range: 53 to 80 years) with probable DAT according to current diagnostic criteria (NINCDS-ADRDA) (2). Flash and pattern-reversal visually evoked potentials were within the normal range. Thus any precortical cause of visual dysfunction was excluded. Neuropsychological testing included the Mini-Mental State examination (MMSE) to establish the severity of dementia (mean score: 19.7, range 9 to 27). Patients were investigated with PET of ^{18}F-2-fluoro-2-deoxyglucose (FDG) for measurement of rCMRGl, and visual information processing was evaluated psychometrically by the fragmented picture test (FPT) (3), which is a combined perception and memory task.

Results. Reduction of the rCMRGl of the primary visual field (area 17), significantly correlating (p=0.03) with impairment of the perception task of the FBT demonstrated involvement of primary sensory cortex in the pathological changes in most patients with DAT. Further significant correlations between the memory part of the FBT and both the MMSE (p=0.04) and the rCMRGl of the secondary visual fields (area 18 and 19) (p=0.008) were found. These finding demonstrate, that impairment of perception due to affection of the primary visual cortex may occur in DAT in addition to disturbance of more complex functions which are related to dementia severity and reductions of rCMRGl in association areas.

References.
1. Mendez FM, Tomsak, RL, Remler B (1990) Disorders of the visual system in Alzheimer's disease. J Clin Neuro-ophthalmol 10:62-69
2. McKhann G, Drachman D, Folstein M, Katzman R, Price D, Stadlan EM (1984) Clinical diagnosis of Alzheimer's disease: report of the NINCDS-ADRDA work group under the auspices of Department of Health and Human Services Task Force on Alzheimer's disease. Neurology 19:939-944
3. Kessler J, Schaaf A, Mielke R (1992) Fragmentierter Bildertest. Hogrefe, Göttingen Toronto Berlin, in press.

34

QUANTITATIVE ANALYSIS OF EYE MOVEMENTS IN SENILE DEMENTIA OF ALZHEIMER TYPE

A. Moser, J. Olschinka and D. Kömpf
Department of Neurology, Medical University, Ratzeburger Allee 160, D-2400 Lübeck, F.R.G.

Ten patients with senile dementia of Alzheimer type (SDAT; mean age 68 ± 5 years) and 12 normal controls (C, mean age 73 ± 7 years) were recruited to measure visually guided reflexive saccades, exploring and searching saccades as well as smooth pursuit eye movements (SPEM). The diagnosis of Alzheimer's dementia were based upon DSM-III criteria. Eye movements were recorded by infrared reflection technique. The infrared light was reflected from each iris plane onto a linear array of 1,024 photo diodes. The analog data resulted were displayed and digitized at 200 Hz. An on-line microcomputer system was used to control stimuli and to analyze the eye movement data according to Katz et al. [1].

In the first session reflexive saccades were induced by moving the target horizontally in square wave patterns with amplitudes of 14°, unpredictable in frequency and direction. There was no significant differences in amplitudes (SDAT 14.3°, C 14.1°), peak velocity (SDAT 426°/s, C 427°/s), and latencies (SDAT 205 ms, C 181 ms) comparing both groups. In the second session smooth pursuit was elicited by moving the target triangularly in a trajectory with frequency of 0.25 Hz and velocity of 15°/s. The maximal amplitudes were 15°. No significant difference in SPEM gain could be demonstrated. The group means of gain were 0.79 in SDAT compared to 0.85 of the normal subjects.

In session 3, the subjects were required to explore the whole target-screen. The first screen consisted of a 64 randomized coloured square pattern (red, blue, yellow, and green, 4x4 cm in size each) resulting in a visual field of 20° x 10°, horizontal (h) x vertical (v) [2]. In the next experiment five horizontally arranged series of 17 letters each, with horizontal and vertical letter distance of 2.5° were presented. The whole visual field was 40° x 10°, h x v, and the subjects were required to search the letters "A". In the third experiment a kitchen scene (20° x 10°, h x v) was presented and the subjects were instructed to scan the scene. In these experiments, the numbers of internally triggered saccades were significantly reduced in patients with SDAT when compared to control, however, without differences of quantitative parameters of the saccades. The mean intersaccadic fixation times were increased almost 2 fold in comparison to control. Since in all experiments of session 3 the results were rather similar, we suggest that impaired systematic, voluntary, internally organized scanning of the environment is due to perceptional or attentional deficits in patients with senile dementia of Alzheimer type.

References

1. Katz B, Mueller K, Helme H (1987)
   Binocular eye movement recording with CCD arrays
   Neuro-ophthalmology 7: 81-91
2. Moser A, Kömpf D (1990)
   Unilateral visual exploration deficit in a frontal lobe lesion.
   Neuro-ophthalmology 10: 39-44

35

VISUAL RESULTS AFTER TRANSSPHENOIDAL OPERATION OF PITUITARY ADENOMAS

H. Seyer, R. Fahlbusch, *M. Küchle

Department of Neurosurgery and *Department of Ophthalmology,
University of Erlangen-Nuremberg,
FRG

Patients with pituitary adenomas present in about 20 % of cases with a chiasmal syndrome. The extent of ophthalmological disturbances widely depends on the height of the adenoma, its symmetrical or asymmetrical suprasellar extension and its consistency.

In about 90 % of our patients, the adenoma is operated on by a transsphenoidal approach. We present the ophthalmological results of 50 patients with chiasmal syndrome, who were operated by a transsphenoidal procedure between 1988 and 1990. They were reexamined 1 to 2 weeks after the operation, after 3 months, and again after 1 year. In 42 cases it was the first operative procedure. In these patients, none showed visual deterioration. 57 % improved, and 40 % showed normalization. Visual function (visual acuity and visual fields) was evaluated according to criteria of the Deutsche Ophthalmologische Gesellschaft (DOG). About half of the patients showed good visual results already a few weeks after the operation. However, improvement may be seen even after one year.

In comparison to preceding series, visual improvement has been achieved in a greater amount of patients. This is due to sophisticated microsurgical means, and also modern sensitive ophthalmological examinations which allow early diagnosis, e.g. red-free photographs of the nerve fibre layer. The visual prognosis has to be judged more reservedly in secondary operations, in patients with advanced age, and after transcranial procedure.

36

ARACHNOIDITIS OF THE OPTIC NERVE WITH LATE ONSET OPTIC ATROPHY AFTER HEAD INJURY - A CASE REPORT

Oberwittler C°, Awe B*, König H-J+, Masur H°, Gerding H*, Schuierer G#, Brune GG°
Dept. of Neurology°, Ophthalmology*, Neurosurgery+ and Radiology#, Westfälische Wilhelms-Universität, Albert-Schweitzer-Str.33, W-4400 Münster, Germany.

Traumatic lesions of the optic nerve with loss of vision and visual field defects as an immediate complication of head injuries are usually caused by direct or indirect compression, e.g. by bone fragments or nerve sheet haemorrhages within the orbita or within the optic canal. There have been only few reports about chronic arachnoiditis with optic atrophy as a late sequela of blunt head trauma. Case report: a 22 year old man noticed an impaired visual acuity of his left eye one year after a blunt head trauma (left parieto-occipital fracture and small right fronto-temporal contusion). Two months later the vision of his right eye started to deteriorate. Within 10 months the visual acuity declined to 0,05 on his left eye and 0,2 on the right side. On the left side an optic atrophy with absence of capillary filling in the retinal angiogram and a central scotoma was found. No visual evoked potential (VEP) could be recorded on the left side, the P100 latency was 103 msec on the right. The CSF was normal, no metabolic abnormalities could be found. The family history was negative. The patient did not drink alcohol regularly. The magnetic resonance tomography (MRT) revealed a relatively small diameter of the intracranial portion of both optic nerves. No other abnormalities could be detected, esp. no signs of demyelinating disease of the central white matter. A neurosurgical operation was performed using a transtemporal approach. The arachnoida of the intracranial part of the optic nerves was thickened and firm. After dissecting the arachnoidea on both sides the left optic nerve appeared atrophic but no compression was seen. Following the operation the deficits gradually improved until a nearly complete recovery. Three years later the visual acuity was 0.8 on the left side and 1.0 on the right. A small paracentral scotoma was present on the left. The VEP of the left eye could be recorded with a P100 latency of 107 msec, the right was unchanged (103 msec). Discussion: The intraoperative findings and the postoperative course can be seen as evidence that the progressive optic atrophy in this patient was caused by posttraumatic arachnoiditis of the intracranial part of the optic nerve. Posttraumatic arachnoditis with late onset optic atrophy has only rarely been reported (1). An impaired microcirculation of the optic nerve is thought to be an important factor in the pathogenesis of posttraumatic optic atrophy associated with arachnoiditis (2). Chronic arachnoiditis of the intracranial optic nerve should be included in the differential diagnosis of optic atrophy in patients with a previous history of head trauma. The neurosurgical intervention in the described patient was followed by a nearly complete recovery and should therefore be considered in similar instances even if no abnormality can be seen on MRT.

1. Brihaye J (1981) Transcranial decompression of the optic nerve after trauma. In: Samii M, Janetta PJ (ed) The cranial nerves. Springer, Berlin Heidelberg New York, pp 116-124

2. Gjerris F (1976) Traumatic lesions of the visual pathways. In: Vinken PJ, Bruyn GW (Ed) Handbook of clinical neurology, North Holland Publishing Co., Amsterdam Oxford, Vol.24, pp 27-58

37

Vertical gaze paralysis as prominent feature of Niemann-Pick disease type C (NP-C)

TRABERT W [1], GRUNDMANN M [2]

[1] University of Saarland, Department of Psychiatry (Head: Prof K Wanke)
[2] University of Saarland, Department of Neurology (Head: Prof K Schimrigk)
D-6650 Homburg/Saar
Germany

Niemann-Pick disease is an autosomal recessive lipid storage disease with hepato-spleno-megaly and accumulation of sphingomyelin and other lipids in liver, spleen and bone marrow. According to the activity of sphingomyelinase, Niemann-Pick disease is differentiated into the forms with marked deficiency of sphingomyelinase activity (type A, B and F) and those forms with only slight reduced or even normal sphingomyelinase activity (type C, D and E).

Niemann-Pick type C (NP-C) can be subdivided into 3 distinguishable phenotypes according to the age of onset and the mode of progression: (1) an early-onset, rapidly progressive form associated with severe hepatic dysfunction and psychomotor retardation during childhood and later with vertical gaze paralysis, ataxia, spasticity and dementia; (2) a delayed-onset, slowly progressive form with mild intellectual impairment, supranuclear vertical gaze paralysis and ataxia, later associated with dementia, seizures and extrapyramidal signs; (3) a late-onset form (adolescence or even adulthood) with very slow progression.

Diagnosis of NP-C is verified biochemically by demonstration of markedly impaired intracellular cholesterol esterification rates in fibroblast cultures.

Detection of heterozygotous subjects, and thereby genetic advice, is possible by the same method, because heterozygotous subjects have an intermediate range of esterification rates compared to affected patients and controls.

We observed a 45-year-old male patient who was firstly diagnosed suffering from hepatosplenomegaly during childhood. Except thrombocytopenia, there were no pathological features. Psychomotor development during childhood and adolescence was completely normal, and he made a successful apprenticeship as an electrician.

By the age of 27 he underwent a simple operation and was seen preoperatively by a specialist for internal diseases who found neurologically only a very mild dysarthric language.

He was firstly admitted to a neurological department in the age of 35 because of etiologically unclear intellectual impairment, ataxia, dysarthric speech, choreo-athetoid movements of the upper extremities, and vertical gaze paresis. Cranial computed tomography revealed no atrophy. Visual evoked potentials as well as motoric and sensoric nerve conduction velocities were within normal limits. EEG was not pathologically altered. In the bone marrow macrophages and lipophages were seen suspicious for a lipid storage disease. Activity of lysosomal enzymes (including sphingomyelinase) was normal.

His daughter of 2.5 years was admitted at the same time to a pediatric hospital suffering from splenomegaly without any neurologic deficits (her mother was born in Romania, and there was no consanguinity with the family of our patient); a diagnosis of possible Niemann-Pick disease was made.

All the patient's symptoms showed a slow but continuous progression: By the age of 43 he had firstly a psychomotor and secondary generalized epileptic seizure and intellectual impairment was severe (dementia). Neuro-ophthalmological status yielded a severe supranuclear vertical gaze paralysis. Cranial computed tomography revealed global atrophy with infratentorial accentuation. NMR did not yield further information. Now, visual evoked potentials showed delayed latencies, and motoric and sensoric nerve conduction velocities (n. suralis and n. peroneus) were diminished. Somatosensoric evoked potentials (n. medianus) revealed a delay of the late central peaks.

The daughter did not develop any neurological symptoms till the age of 12. In her bone marrow sea-blue histiozytes were found.

Fibroblast cultures of our patient as well as of his daughter revealed a very marked deficiency of intracellular cholesterol esterification in the daughter and a not as much pronounced deficiency in the father.

Interestingly, a now 46-year-old sister of our patient suffers from an etiologically unknown and slowly progressive dysarthric disorder and gait disturbances. Although we do not know anything definite about this clinical picture, it may be supposed that she might be affected by this disease, too.

The unique feature of this family is the fact that without any doubt father and daughter are suffering both from Niemann-Pick disease type C. Normally, this disorder is transmitted in an autosomal recessive mode, and affection of father and daughter simultaneously are not found. There are two possible explanations for our exceptional findings: (1) In the case of this family we have to consider an autosomal dominant inheritance, or (2), if one wants to maintain the concept of a recessive transmission: both the parents of our patient were heterozygotous and therefore clinically not affected, and our patient (homozygotous) married again a heterozygotous carrier with the subsequent risk of 50 % for their children to develop the same disorder.

Literature:

1. Fink JK, Filling-Katz MR, Sokol J, Cogan DG, Pikus A, Sonies B, Soong B, Pentchev PG, Comly ME, Brady RO, Barton NW (1989) Clinical spectrum of Niemann-Pick disease type C. Neurology 39: 1040-1049
2. Vanier MT, Pentchev P, Rodriguez-Lafrasse C, Rousson R (1991) Niemann-Pick disease type C: an update. J Inher Metab Dis 14: 580-595

38

OPTIC ATAXIA DUE TO HEMISPHERIC LESIONS - CORRELATION WITH OCULOMOTOR AND VISUO-SPATIAL DEFICITS

S. Drescher, W. Heide and D. Kömpf
Dept. of Neurology, Medical University, Ratzeburger Allee 160, DW-2400 Lübeck, GERMANY

Optic ataxia (OA) is an inaccuracy of visually elicited, goal-directed hand and arm movements, not related to basic motor, somatosensory or visual deficits. Since its first descirption by Balint in 1909, it has been reported several times following bilateral or unilateral hemispheric lesions, always including the posterior parietal lobe. The mechanism of OA is still a matter of discussion. It cannot generally be explained as a feature of visuo-spatial disorientation, because OA was found also in patients without visuo-spatial deficits. Most authors considered OA as a visuo-motor disconnection syndrome, caused by disruption of fibers that process visual information from the occipital to the frontal lobes. If this is true, it should be possible that also isolated lesions of more anterior brain regions lead to OA, but this has not been reported so far. There is, however, evidence from single unit recordings in monkeys as well as from cerebral blood flow and positron emission tomography studies in humans that the posterior parietal cortex itself is involved in visuo-motor coordination, not only the underlying white matter. As the posterior parietal cortex has multimodal functions, including ocular motor, visuo-vestibular and visuo-spatial, we investigated how deficits of these functions correlate with OA.

Among 10 patients with OA, 8 had unilateral lesions of the posterior parietal lobe (7 right and 1 left hemispheric), always including the cortex around the intraparietal sulcus and - in the right hemispheric cases - the adjacent upper part of the angular gyrus. Two patients had extraparietal lesions, one in the posterior limb of the right internal capsule, due to ischemia in the territory of the posterior choroidal artery, and the other in the fronto-temporal white matter, just lateral to the caput of the caudate nucleus, thus being the first reported case of OA due to an isolated anterior hemispheric lesion. Lesions had been caused by cerebral ischemia (7 cases), hemorrhage (1 case) or tumour surgery (2 cases), 0.5 to 72 (mean 13.6) months prior to examination. None of the patients had manifest hemiparesis, proprioceptive or visual field deficits (except the posteror choroidal case with homonymous hemianopia).

Neuropsychological testing revealed visuo-spatial disorientation and constructive apraxia in 3 cases and latent or manifest contralateral visual hemineglect in 5 of the right parietal cases and in the patient with the posterior capsular lesion. Only those patients showed a prominent "visual field effect" of OA, which means that OA involved both hands, but was much more obvious for targets in the contralateral visual hemifield. Correspondingly, the "hand effect" with predominant involvement of the contralateral hand for targets in both hemifields was more pronounced in the fronto-temporal case and in the remaining parietal cases where lesions extended more towards the superior parietal lobulus. The subjective straight ahead, as assessed psychophysically by directing a laser target in darkness was shifted into the ipsilateral hemifield in only 4 cases (all right parietal lesions), so it cannot account for dysmetric arm movements in most of the OA patients.

Different types of saccadic and pursuit eye movements were examined using infrared reflection oculography. Exploratory eye movements showed a directional bias towards the ipsilateral hemifield only in the 6 cases with latent or manifest visual hemineglect, but were normal in the others. Compared to 30 age-matched normal adults, visually guided and memory-guided saccades had significantly prolonged latencies and reduced amplitudes in 4 out of 7 right parietal cases and in the posterior capsular case. Other deficits like reduced gain of smooth pursuit and optokinetic nystagmus with ipsiversive stimulation were found in 50 to 70% of the OA patients, asymmetries of vestibular nystagmus or mild contralaterally beating spontaneous nystagmus in 30%. But as these deficits were not present in the remaining cases including the fronto-temporal lesion, they did not really correlate with OA.

In conclusion, the typical site of lesions causing OA is the posterior parietal cortex around the intraparietal sulcus, with a dominance of the right hemisphere. Exceptionally, disruption of its efferent projection through the posterior internal capsule or of the visuo-motor projection towards the frontal lobes can cause OA. The disorder cannot generally be attributed to visuo-spatial or ocular motor deficits being coincidentally found only in right parietal cases, correlating with the presence of a "visual field effect". Other hemispheric lesions, however, rather cause a different type of OA, with predominance of the "hand effect", usually not being associated with disorders of eye movements or visuo-spatial perception.

39

THREE-DIMENSIONAL PROPERTIES OF THE HUMAN VESTIBULO-OCULAR REFLEX DURING SINUSOIDAL ROTATION

D. Fischer, M. Fetter, D.Tweed[*], H.Misslisch, E.Koenig. Department of Neurology, University of Tübingen, Germany; [*]Department of Physiology, University of Western Ontario, London, Ontario, Canada.

The vestibuloocular reflex (VOR) helps to stabilize the retinal image by rotating the eyes to compensate for movements of the head. In the past, the VOR has usually been studied 1-dimensionally and characterized by its *gain*, which is the number g relating VOR input (head velocity, h) to output (eye velocity, e): $e = g \times h$. In reality, VOR input and output are 3-component vectors: the angular velocity vectors of the head and eye. The 3-dimensional generalization of the gain is a 3×3 matrix G such that $e = G \times h$. The 9 components of this matrix describe the dependence of all 3 components of eye velocity on all 3 components of head velocity. Using a new 3-D motor-driven rotating chair and a 3-D magnetic search-coil system, we determined the gain matrices for the human VOR under various stimulus conditions.

Six normal human subjects were rotated sinusoidally in darkness with the head at the center of rotation in a computer-controlled chair at .3 Hz, maximum speed 37°/s, about the naso-occipital, interaural, and body-vertical axes as well as in the canal planes, and with the axes earth-vertical (Otolith input Constant: OC) or earth-horizontal (Otolith input Variable: OV). Subjects looked at an imagined target straight ahead. Head and left eye position were measured using 3-D search coils, and 3-D angular velocities of eye in head and of head in space were calculated from the coil signals and information about the chair's rotation. VOR matrices were computed by relating instantaneous eye and head velocity vectors over 2 cycles of rotation (6.7 s) by linear approximation using a least squares method.

Rotations around at least 3 axes, not all lying in a single plane relative to the body, are required to compute a VOR matrix. If a single gain matrix faithfully depicts the input-output characteristics of the VOR, then the computed matrix should be the same for any combination of axes. Matrices were calculated for rotations about the major body axes -- either with all axes earth-vertical (OC), earth-horizontal (OV), or "natural" (NAT i.e. pitch and roll about an earth-horizontal and yaw about an earth-vertical axis) -- and for rotations in the semicircular canal planes, again under "natural" conditions. Calculated matrices were almost identical (diagonal elements: torsion about .4, vertical and horizontal about .65 - .7) for the 2 sets of body axes, indicating that a single matrix depicts VOR responses to stimuli about all these axes. There were also no significant differences between OC, OV and NAT matrices, indicating that the otolith organs have little influence on the VOR at the stimulation frequency used. In all cases, off-diagonal matrix elements (representing crosstalk in the VOR) were minimal.

This study was supported by the Deutsche Forschungsgemeinschaft, SFB 307, A2. Douglas Tweed was a Fellow of the Medical Research Council of Canada.

40

Clinical Application of Continuous Infrared-Pupillography (IRPG)

Katja Lortz and W.H.Zangemeister
Neurological University Clinic Hamburg, FRG

Alexandridis (1971) and Müller-Jensen (1975) reported a reliable clinical method to measure the phasic pupillary light reflex using an infrared reflection technique. We modified and extended this method to measure additionally continuous sinusoidal pupillary responses between 0.02 Hz and 0.9 Hz. 20 healthy subjects and 20 neurological patients (11 M.S., 6 cerebellar atrophies, 3 diabetic neuropathies) were compared. Besides the re-evaluation for monocular stimulation and recordings of earlier normal values of latency, response amplitude, velocity of constriction and redilation we looked particularly for phase lags or leads using the continuous IRPG.

M.S. patients showed significant latency increases together with relatively constant phase lags, however without clear effects on response amplitudes. The cerebellar patients demonstrated a highly variable phase that interchanged between lag and lead, as described by Hultborn et al. 1978, with mostly decreased response amplitudes. The diabetic patients with polyneuropathy did not show any effects on response amplitude, but phase lags especially for fast frequencies.

Recently a model of the pathways controlling the size and frequency response of the human pupil was presented by Krenz et al. 1985. Simulations of the effects of some well known pupillary abnormalities (Stark 1959) and of drugs analytically demonstrated the workings of the underlying internal processes. Comparison of clinical findings using particularly continuous IRPG with model simulations will help to improve the fine diagnostic of pupillary disturbances as a valuable sign of underlying neurological diseases.

References:
1.AlexandridisE (1971) Pupillographie: Anwendungsmöglichkeiten als objektive Untersuchungsmethode. Hüthig, Heidelberg
2.Müller-JensenA(1975) Anwendungsmöglichkeiten der Infrarot-Reflexpupillographie in der Neurologie. Nervenarzt 46: 281-284
3.HultbornH, MoriK, TsukaharaN (1978) Cerebellar influence on parasympathetic neurones innervating intra-ocular muscles.
4.KrenzW, RobinM, BarezS, StarkL (1985) Abnormal human pupil. IEEE TransBME:32 817-825
5.StarkL (1959) Stability, oscillations and noise in the human pupil servomechanism. Proc.IRE 47: 1925-1939

41

ANTICIPATION OF A VISUAL TARGET MODIFIES THE VESTIBULO-OCULAR REFLEX

C. Moschner and W. H. Zangemeister
Dept. of Neurology , University Hospital Hamburg-Eppendorf
2000 Hamburg 20 , Germany

Fast orienting eye-head movements towards a peripheral visual target consist naturally of an eye saccade and synkinetic head trajectory. The latter provides an input to the angular vestibulo-ocular reflex (VOR). Prior studies in humans show that the intrasaccadic VOR gain decreased with large target displacements. The purpose of our study was to examine the effects of anticipation on the eye-head coordination and the intrasaccadic VOR gain.

Five healthy human subjects were tested under four experimental paradigms represented different levels of target shift predictability. Sequences of horizontal target steps were presented with (a) a constant frequency (0.5 Hz) and constant amplitude (of 20,40,60 or 80 deg), (b) randomized frequencies (0.2-1.2 Hz) while the amplitudes remained constant,(c) a constant frequency and a random sequence of varying amplitudes (10-80 deg) or (d) a combination of randomized frequencies and amplitudes. All paradigms were tested with the subject's head fixed in a center position or during fast voluntary head movements. The stimuli consisted of bright green LED lights on a semicircular screen 1.2 from the center of the head.

Horizontal EOG signals of both eyes were averaged to gain the eye position. The horizontal head position was measured by a high resolution-angular potentiometer that was rigidly linked to the light weight-helmet. Both signals were added to calculate the gaze position (eye-in-space). EOG calibrations were repeated every 10-15 min with an accuracy of <1.0 deg. All subjects show anticipatory gaze movements (latency < 100 msec) in response to the highly predictable target paradigm (a) whereas randomized target steps (b-d) let to typical latencies of +150 to +250 msec. Compared to the saccades in the head fixed-condition, the gaze latencies and accuracies of orienting eye-head shifts were about the same in the corresponding paradigms.

However, in all subjects the peak gaze velocities of the combined movements were significantly faster than pure saccades (p<0.01, t-test) when the target displacement was highly predictable and exceeded 30 deg of amplitude. In two subjects eye-head shifts were significantly faster in the random frequency paradigm (b), but the velocity increase was comparatively smaller. No such velocity effect was observed during the highly randomized trials (c + d).

While tracking the highly predictable target steps (a) the head movements started 40-220 msec before the saccade resulting in significantly larger amplitude and velocity of the head during the saccade whereas in randomized trials (b-d) the saccades led the head trajectory by a time interval that correlated positively with the level of randomization. When the intrasaccadic VOR gain was calculated for the largest gaze shifts of about 80 deg , the anticipatory eye-head movements in the highly predictable target paradigm (a) showed an averaged VOR gain reduction of about 40% compared to responses in the random frequency-paradigm (b). Due to the relatively large standard deviations of these gain values, the reduction was statistically significant only in three out of the five subjects (p<0.05, t-test).

We concluded that highly predictable target patterns allow human subjects to preprogram time optimized eye-head movements. With respect to pure saccades, the early initiation of synkinetic head movements resulted in a significant velocity increase and reduced duration. Aditionally, the intrasaccadic VOR gain was modified in advance to maintain the gaze accuracy. The efficacy of a combined eye-head movement was related to the required movement amplitude. A significant velocity increase was observed during target steps beyond 30 deg. If a successful anticipation was prevented by randomization of the target, head contribution to the overall gaze displacement was significantly reduced, possibly because of relatively slow peripheral head mechanisms. The VOR *gain* was consequently higher in randomized target trials.

42

Optic Neuritis – a Disease Entity or Symptom of Multiple Sclerosis

Rüttinger H., Krekel Ch., Schimrigk K.
University of Saarland, Department of Neurology
D-6650 Homburg/Saar

The nosologic classification of optic neuritis (ON) is subject of controvers discussion and depends on selection criteria, the quality of diagnostic techniques and the length of the catamnestic period. F.e. more than 20 ys can pass between the first manifestation and the next relapse of multiple sclerosis (MS). Reports about the percentage of patients which develope MS in the course of an ON vary from 8 to 91 %.

81 patients with a clear history of acute ON were studied by VEP, investigation of CSF (including isoelectric focusing and quantitative measurement of albumin and IgG) and cranial MRI. Other causes for reduced visual acuity or delayed VEP latencies (f.e. vascular or toxic disorders) were carefully excluded. The data of ON patients were compared with clinical and CSF-data of 419 MS patients of our hospital.

72 of the 81 patients suffered from retrobulbar neuritis (RBN, retrolaminar localisation), 9 patients showed the picture of a papillitis. The localisation of the inflammatory process was somehow related to the number of abnormal findings in the paraclinical investigations: most patients with papillitis had normal or slightly abnormal CSF and MRI (6/9 neg. oligoclonal bands (OB), 5/9 normal cell count; 7/9 no lesions on MRI, 1x one periventricular lesion, 1x a few small lesions). On the contrary, most of the patients with RBN had abnormal results in the supplementary investigations (f.e. 68/72 pos. OB). Focusing on first clinical manifestations only, already more than 90% had pos. OB and ≈ 2/3 had disseminated lesions on MRI. If ON was at least the second exacerbation (n = 25), OB were always positive.

Comparing the data of ON-patients with those of MS-patients (especially of the relapsing-remitting type) we found an identical CSF profile, the same age of onset of the disease and the same predominance of the female sex. Even the frequent occurence of exacerbations in spring and summer is a corresponding feature in ON and MS.

From our data it can be concluded, that retrobulbar neuritis is a typical symptom of MS, which however cannot always be diagnosed with definite certainty at the time of ON. In contrast papillitis only sometimes belongs to the spectrum of MS symptoms, a fact which has great prognostic importance.

43

Visual deficits in Multiple Sclerosis are due to a lesion of the magnocellular pathway

H. Herbst, P. Thier and J. Dichgans
Department of Neurology, Hoppe-Seyler-Str. 3
7400 Tübingen, Germany

Increases in the latency of visual evoked potentials (VEP) in multiple sclerosis (MS) reflect demyelinating lesions of the optic pathways. These lesions can occur without subjective impairment of vision or any pathological results in traditional visual tests. Work done by Regan et al. [1] suggests that mainly magnocellular parts of the visual system are affected in MS. Therefore, specific examination of magnocellular functions would be helpful in revealing visual deficits. In order to test this hypothesis we compared the results of two tests of the magnocellular system (Contrast Reduced Letter Test, CRL-test; Motion Defined Letter Test [2], MDL-test) with data derived from traditional visual acuity tests (Snellen charts) and latency changes of VEPs (reversed checkerboard pattern) in 11 patients with MS.

The *CRL-test* is based on the presentation of contrast reduced optotypes (4 % and 11 % contrast) otherwise identical to those used in conventional Snellen charts. The *MDL-test* utilizes optotypes that are made visible by dots moving in and outside the letter at equal speeds in opposite directions. The detection threshold for the detection of motion defined letters was defined as the velocity at which subjects produced 75 % correct optotype identifications. Motion-defined letters were also utilized to measure *motion defined visual acuity*.

43 % of all eyes examined presented a significant increase of VEP latency (see figure: region c+d). 78% of these cases (region d) showed elevated velocity thresholds in the MDL test (mean of patients 3.3 times larger than upper limit of control sample), and 66 % also exhibited pathological acuity changes as determined by Snellen charts. Measurement of visual acuity using solely motion defined optotypes identical to those in the MDL-test revealed deficits in 89 % of the patients with pathological VEP latencies.

The remainder of eyes tested (57 %) exhibited no increased VEP latency (region a+b) despite definite diagnosis of MS. 50% of these cases (region b) showed disturbances in motion detection in the MDL-test while only 8% exhibited a reduction of visual acuity as measured by conventional Snellen charts. Utilizing the CRL-test abnormalities were detected in half of the eyes that tested normally using the MDL-test. The ad-

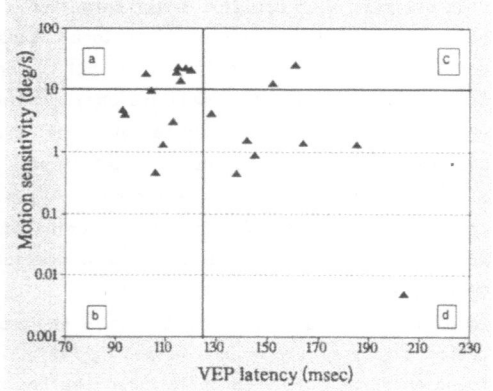

a= normal VEP and normal motion sensitiviy
b=normal VEP, pathological motion sensitivity
c= pathological VEP, normal motion sensitivity
d=pathological VEP and pathol. motion sensitivity

dition of the CRL-test led to a significant increase in detection of abnormalities in patients who exhibited no increase of VEP latency.

Our results emphasize once again that pathological VEP latencies do not represent functionally insignificant lesions. The deficits in visual function discussed here could lead to severe impairment of visuomotor performance such as driving capability. Moreover our results indicate that a psychophysical examination has the potential to reveal lesions of the visual system even in patients with normal VEPs and thus might help to contribute to the diagnosis of MS.

[1] *Regan D, Kothe AC and Sharpe JA* (1991) Recognition of motion-defined shapes in patients with multiple sclerosis and optic neuritis. Brain: 114, 1129-1155

[2] *Regan D & Hong XH* (1990) Visual acuity for optptypes made visible by relative motion. Optometry and Vision Science: 67, 49-55

Supported by DFG: KFG Neuroopthalmologie

44

Cerebrospinal fluid parameters in patients with optic neuritis

Sigrid Scharein, Christiane Hartard and Klaus Kunze
Clinic of Neurology, University of Hamburg, FRG

Introduction

Although unilateral optic neuritis may be caused by multiple sclerosis (MS) in about 40 - 60% of cases, it is still doubtful whether there is a realistic risk of developing MS after initial monosymptomatic optic neuritis. About 20% of patients with a diagnosis of MS never develop a clinical optic neuritis [for review see e.g. 1]. Since several authors report a higher risk of developing MS in the case of abnormal cerebrospinal fluid (CSF) parameters, we analysed CSF parameters in patients with monosymptomatic optic neuritis and no clinical signs of multiple sclerosis.

Method

During the years 1982 - 91, lumbar punctures were performed in 98 patients (age 14 - 58, 34 ± 10.9) with isolated optic neuritis. Cerebrospinal fluid parameters were evaluated by the blood - CSF barrier model of Reiber and Felgenhauer [3]. We describe the distribution of the different CSF - parameters statistically and analyse the relations between oligoclonal bands, locally synthesised immunoglobulins and cytology.

Results

Locally synthesised immunoglobulin fractions in the CSF were found in 60 of 88 patients (68%) for which data were available. Most of them had locally synthesised immunoglobulin G (52%), immunoglobulin M was observed in 9% of the patients and immunoglobulin A in 7%. As expected, an increased quotient of albumin (IgG_{CSF} / IgG_{serum}) as indicator of a broken blood - CSF barrier occurred only in 4 patients (5%).

Oligoclonal immunoglobulin in isoelectric focusing could be detected in 66% of the patients. In 62% the oligoclonal bands were observed only in the CSF and 4% had parallel bands in CSF and serum as a sign of a systemic alteration. In 34% there were no oligoclonal bands detectable. Cytological data were available in 62 patients. 25 of them (40%) exhibited a pleocytosis of 12/3 - 186/3 (20/3 ± 28/3). Normal CSF - parameters were seen only in 25 of 98 patients.

Discussion

In our sample of patients with monosymptomatic optic neuritis without clinical diagnosis of multiple sclerosis we found a relative high percentage of locally synthesised immunoglobulins (68%). Also the percentage of oligoclonal bands in CSF (66%) was higher than that reported in the literature. Martinelli et al. [2], for example, detected oligoclonal bands in the CSF in 46% of 43 patients with an initial monosymptomatic optic neuritis. The prognostic relevance of the observed pathological alterations in CSF parameters need to be determined in a follow-up study.

References

1. Kelly R (1985) Clinical aspects of multiple sclerosis. In: Koetsier JC (ed) Handbook of Clinical Neurology, Vol. 3. (47): Demyelinating Diseases. Elsevier, Amsterdam, pp 49-78
2. Martinelli V, Comi G, Filippi M, Poggi A, Colombo B, Rodegher M, Scotti G, Triulzi F, Canal N (1991) Paraclinical tests in acute-onset optic neuritis: basal data and results of a short follow-up. Acta Neurol Scand 84: 231 - 236
3. Reiber HO, Felgenhauer K (1987) Protein transfer at the cerebrospinal fluid barrier and the quantitation of the humoral immune response within the central nervous system. Clin Chim Acta 163: 319-328

45

OPTHALMOLOGIC SIGNS IN PATIENTS WITH INTERNAL CAROTID ARTERY DISSECTION

Sievers, C.; Knappertz, V.; Rothacher, G.; Krämer, G.
Dpt. of Neurology; University of Mainz, Germany

Introduction

Internal carotid artery dissection (ICAD) has become an increasingly recognized cause of central neurologic deficit (CND), lower cranial nerve palsy, neck pain and Horner's syndrome (HS) especially in the young. The aim of this study was to analyse the occurrence of peripheral and central neurologic deficits with respect to a possible correlation with the site of the vascular lesion.

Patients and Methods

Thirty consecutive patients (17 male, 13 female; median age 46, range 28-64 years) with acute spontaneous or traumatic unilateral (n = 28) or bilateral (n = 2) ICAD were identified with initial duplex sonography and confirmed by intraarterial angiography (n = 28) or magnetic resonance immaging (n = 6).

Results

Ophthalmo-neurologic symptoms were observed in 9/32 ICAD. They consisted of 8 partial HS, i.e. without change of sweating in the face, and 1 ischemic optic neuropathy. One patient showed a Collet-Sicard syndrome. Pure CND was caused by 21/32 ICAD corresponding to the ipsilateral hemisphere (TIA, stroke, ischemic optic neuropathy). Of 8 patients with HS 5 initially complained of pain in the ipsilateral neck of which 3 also had a CND. Two patients presented with HS and CND but without pain. Only 1 patient showed a HS without CND or pain. In each of 2 patients with bilateral ICAD one side was asymptomatic.

In patients with HS 7/8 vascular lesions were in or reached the proximal portion of the ICA: 4 ICADs appeared as tapered occlusions arising from the ICA origin, 3 as proximal ICA stenoses, and 1 as distal stenosis at the skull basis.
In patients without HS 7 tapered occlusions, 3 proximal ICA stenoses, and 12 distal lesions were found.

Discussion and Conclusions

HS is a frequently occuring clinical sign in patients with ICAD (1). An isolated partial HS can be the only clinical sign. The possibility of ICAD causing interruption of the ascending postsynaptic sympathetic fibres adjacent to the ICA, of the superior cervical ganglion, or of the carotid nerve has to be considered in these patients. Duplex sonography by itself was able to detect 84% of ICAD in our series and should be used as a screening method. Our results suggest that patients with ICAD and HS tend to have more lesions reaching down to the proximal ICA than patients without HS. The relevance of these findings remains uncertain taking into account that the intramural carotid plexus is supposed to take its course in the segment distal to the superior cervical ganglion. These findings may suggest that the more extended lesions reaching from the base of the skull down to the ICA origin indicate a more severe mural disturbance of the distal ICA thus enabling those lesion to cause a postganglionic HS. There are subintimal or subadventitial locations of ICAD. The latter has been proposed to be more frequently associated with HS (2). Further pathological data on the exact intramural localization of the lesion in patients with ICAD and HS as well as sweat and pupil stimulation tests are needed (3).

Literatur:

1. Mokri B, Sundt TM, Hauser OW (1979) Spontaneous internal carotid dissection, hemicrania, and Horner's syndrome. Arch Neurol 36:677-680
2. Hacke W, Hennerici M, Gelmers J, Krämer G (1991) Cerebral Ischemia, 1991 Springer Verlag, Berlin, Heidelberg, New York, p.82
3. Thomson HS, Mensher JH (1971) Adrenergic mydriasis in Horner's syndrome. Am J Ophth 72:472-480

46

Latencies of visually evoked perfusion changes in the posterior cerebral artery territory

J. Klingelhöfer, I. Wittich, D. Sander, B. Conrad

Department of Neurology, Technical University of Munich, Möhlstraße 28, W-8000 München 80

Methods used so far to measure cerebral blood flow (e. g. PET, SPECT) are still too slow to register the dynamics of regulation processes taking place in the order of seconds between neuronal activity and cerebral blood flow. Based on measurements of flow velocity changes, the time courses of these local regulatory processes can be evaluated by means of transcranial Doppler ultrasonography. Up to now, the temporal resolution of velocity changes was linked to the length of a cardiac cycle. By using a pulse-dependent triggering of visual stimuli, the existing rate of resolution resulting from the heart rate was to be extended in the present investigation and the most rapid reaction times between stimulus onset and reactive flow velocity changes were to be determined.

The intracranial flow patterns of the P2-segment of the posterior cerebral artery were investigated after visual stimulation in 12 healthy subjects in response to various visual stimuli. The healthy subjects were seated in complete darkness in a specially developed projection unit during the experiment. Coloured slides with complex pictures projected onto a screen (mean maximum illumination density 61 cd/m², viewing angle of 90° horizontally and 67.4° vertically) served as stimuli. Use of electromagnetic shutters and a quartz-controlled two-level pulse-triggered timer ensured a defined temporal limitation of the stimuli. The stimulus onset was triggered pulse-dependently for precise establishment of the beginning of the reactive velocity changes. In the series of experiments stimulus onset was placed in time using the electronic timer in such a way that the reactive velocity rise occured exactly in the subsequent diastole. Percentage increases of flow velocity due to a reactive decrease of vascular resistance are more pronounced in diastole than in systole, and therefore can be measured better during diastole.

The shortest individual latency between stimulus onset and significant (p<0.05) reactive increase in flow velocity determined in this way varied between 520ms and 1080ms. The average shortest latency of the overall population was 717.3ms±190.9ms.

Comparable latencies were measured in animal experiments for the reactive local rise of the cerebral blood volume in the region of the visual cortex after visual stimulation. These latencies between stimulus onset and significant increase in flow velocity of less than 1 second show that the coupling between neuronal activity changes and reactive perfusion changes and thus the control of cerebral vascular resistance must be regulated via rapidly acting mechanisms. Such a mechanism for regulation of the diameter of cerebral arterioles might be based on the so called cation hypothesis. This hypothesis suggests that the coupling between rised functional activity and rised cerebral blood flow velocity is the local increase in K^+ and H^+ and the local decrease in Ca^{++} in the extracellular fluid surrounding the cerebral arterioles.

47

VISUAL STIMULI AND POSTERIOR CEREBRAL ARTERY BLOOD FLOW

M v.Maravic, Ch. Kessler, A. Böhning, B. Spelsberg, D. Kömpf

Department of Neurology, Medical University of Lübeck, Germany

INTRODUCTION

Specific brain activity is followed within seconds by a metabollically mediated response of cerebral blood flow. In the clinical routine transcranial Dopplersonography (TCD) is used for evaluation of blood flow of the cerebral arteries supplying the activated cortical regions. We were interested in evaluation of the (patho)-physiology of visually induced reagibility (VIR) of blood flow in the PCA to different visual stimuli and visual imagery tasks in normal subjects and patients with PCA-infarctions.

SUBJECTS AND METHODS

32 normal individuals (19 young subjects, mean age 25 + $\underline{3}$ y ; 13 elder subjects, mean age 56 $\pm$ 16 y) without any signs of cerebrovascular disorders were examined as well as 12 patients with by CCT-visible PCA-infarctions in the occipital lobe . 5 patients showed a complete homonymous hemianopsia (4 left-sided and 1 right-sided), 6 had a quadrantanopsia (5 left-sided and 1 right-sided), and one had diffuse multiple lesions in both visual fields. Succesively the left and right PCA were measured using an EME-TC2-64 transcranial Doppler device. A durable 2 MHz probe was installed and the PCA was insonated by transtemporal acces. In a room dimmed from daylight the PCA-baseline flow and it's changes to different stimuli were measured as follow:
1. on-off light stimuli (25 s), 2. color slides, red (25 s), 3. picture slides (25 s), 4: visual imagery tasks (40 s): the subjects were asked to imagine a preferably scene as vividly as possible. Finally the PCA blood flow was stimulated by breathing CO_2 continuously to an endtidal CO_2 of 9 Vol% for calculating the CO_2-dependent dilation reserve.

RESULTS

In normal subjects on-off light stimuli and colored slides produced a mean VIR from 19.5 to 25.2 %. The blood flow increase following complex scenes was significantly higher (25.5 to 30.6 %; p < 0.05). Visual imagery task had no significant effect on the PCA-flow velocities. There were no differences between right or left PCA. In patients with complete homonyous hemianopsia there were no VIR on the affected side; the CO_2-reactivity was significantly reduced when compared to the unaffected side (16.9 $\pm$ 4.5 % vs 55.7 $\pm$ 16.9 %). Patients with quadrantanopsia showed a perceptible decrease of VIR in the on-off-light and colored slide stimuli but not to complex scene stimuli The dilation reserve was slightly reduced in the affected side (about 70% of the normal response).
Visual stimuli had no influence to cerebral blood flow in the middle cerebral artery .

CONCLUSIONS

Depending on the blood supply of both posterior cerebral arteries visual stimuli are only activating the visual cortex. Complex scenes provoced a higher increase of cerebral blood flow than simple light or color stimuli.
We conclude a proportional relation between VIR and the extent of activated cortex (primary visual cortex and association cortex).
The absence of cerebral blood flow response in patients with complete homonymous hemianopsia suggests that visual incuced reagibility depends on a fast metabolic mediated metabolism and therefore also depends on the activity of neurons in the visual cortex.

48

VASOREACTIVITY TO VISUAL STIMULI IN MIGRAINE
M. Carvajal-Lizano, A. Thie
Neurologische Universitätsklinik Hamburg-Eppendorf

Background and objectives:
Previous investigations with transcranial Doppler ultrasound have indicated that an increase of cerebral metabolism due to activating stimuli is rapidly followed by an increase of blood flow velocities (BFV) in the basal cerebral arteries. Migraineurs may exhibit abnormal transcranial ultrasonic features with regard to BFV and vasoreactivity to certain stimuli during the headache-free period. Tests of vasoreactivity could serve as an aid in the diagnosis of migraine, but the most sensitive and feasible test modality remains unknown.

Patients and methods:
We studied changes of BFV after visual stimulation in 25 migraineurs and in 25 age-matched healthy volunteers serving as controls. The posterior cerebral artery was continuously insonated with a fixed 2-MHz probe, and the mean BFV automatically calculated by our Doppler device (TC 2-64 B, EME, Überlingen) every 4 seconds were recorded by hand. Photic stimulation (i.e., strobe light flickering with a frequency of 2 and 10 Hz) and the video of a cartoon were used as visual stimuli. Each test phase lasted for one minute and was applied twice interrupted by rest phases of one minute (with eyes closed). Visual vasoreactivity was calculated from the difference between BFV during test phases compared to rest phases, averaged over the entire period of one minute and over the first 12 seconds (initial response).

Results:
For all tests, visual vasoreactivity was more pronounced in migraineurs than in controls. Differences were statistically significant for the video test for the one-minute response (increase of mean BFV in migraineurs 16.25% vs. 10.05% in controls; p=0.0057) and for photic stimulation for the initial response: migraineurs 10.45% vs. controls 5.23%; p= 0.0031 (2 Hz stimulus); migraineurs 10.03% vs. controls 4.83%; p=0.0034 (10 Hz stimulus).

Conclusions:
Our results suggest abnormal visual vasoreactivity in migraine. The diagnostic value of these findings remain to be determined in a prospective study.

49

Oculomotor Palsy As Leading Sign In Meningovascular Syphilis

Schmitt T., Erbguth F, Taghavy A.
Neurologische Klinik der Universität Erlangen-Nürnberg

In the age of antibiotics neurosyphilis has become so rare in western industrialized countries that despite typical symptoms and signs it is often diagnosed only by serological findings. We present 2 patients with oculomotor palsy caused by meningovascular lues.

Case 1 (52 years, male): admitted because of acute leftsided ptosis. One year history of sleepiness and personality change. 6 months before admission he" dragged" his left leg for some weeks. Although married and father of a son homosexual activities in the past 30 years. No primary lesion remembered. On examination complete oculomotor palsy of the left eye, a discrete leftsided sensomotor hemisyndrome and a positive extensor plantar response on both sides. Neuropsychologic testing revealed mild dementia. Deafness for high frequencies on both sides could be demonstrated by audiometry; caused according to BAEP by a brain stem lesion. CT scan: fusiform dilatation of middle cerebral artery left and several lacunar infarctions in the right thalamus. CSF: 40 cells/cmm (81 % lymphocytes, 2 % plasma cells), protein 190 mg/dl, active syphilis in routine serological tests. TPHA-IgG-liquor-serum-quotient 12,8, 19-S-IgM-FTA-Abs interestingly negative. MRT (T2): leftsided pontomesencephal brain stem infarction in the area of the nerve fascicle of the oculomotor nerve. After daily treatment with 3 x 10 million units Penicillin G-Na IV for two weeks the left eye opened 22 days after admission.

Case 2 (51 years, male): Cause of admission: diplopia, 5 months intermittently, 7 days continously. 5 years before admission primary syphilis (never treated). One year history of enlargement of the right pupil. On examination isolated bilateral incomplete oculomotor palsy with external paresis on the right and internal paresis on the left side. CSF: 92 cells/cmm (86 % lymphocytes, 3 % plasmacells).Serology typical for active neurolues. After two courses of penicillin within 3 months improvement of defects, CSF and serology parameters.

While around 1900 about 50 percent of oculomotor palsys were caused by neurosyphilis, this percentage declined to approximately 1 % today. This reduction is not only a consequence of the dramatic decline of the incidence and prevalence of neurolues after the introduction of penicillin, but also of a decreased frequency of paresis of the third cranial nerve in cases of manifest neurosyphilis from about 34 percent to 5 percent. Today the eighth cranial nerve is most commonly affected cranial nerve in neurolues. Causes of oculomotor nerve damage in neurosyphilis are gummatous and non-gummatous meningitis, interstitial neuritis, thrombosis of vasa nervorum, brain stem infarctions in the area of the nucleus or the nerve fascicle, encephalitis or gummas in the area of the nucleus /nerve fascicle. After literature review we conclude that the relative frequency of oculomotor palsy in cases of neurosyphilis has sharply declined as consequence of the virtual disappearance of gummas, once the leading cause of oculomotor palsy in cerebral syphilis. In a report from the 1950ies penicillin therapy in 5 cases of oculomotor palsy caused by neurosyphilis resulted in complete remissions. Today partial remissions seem to be the rule. Therefore either the main cause of luetic III. nerve palsys has changed (e.g. infarctions instead of gummas) or the efficacy of penicillin has declined.

50

Mitochondriopathies - A special form of ophthalmopareses

Reichmann, H., Gold, R., Beck, A., Maas, J., Seibel, P., and Naumann, M.
Department of Neurology, University of Würzburg, Josef-Schneider-Str.11, D-8700 Würzburg, Germany

Patients with a mitochondriopathy resemble due to their ptosis and ophthalmopareses patients with myasthenia gravis, hypothyreosis, or ocular muscular dystrophy. Our group has extensively characterized 40 such patients with ^{31}P-spectroscopy and bicycle ergometer analyses. Quantitative enzyme analyses in 10 patients with CPEO revealed in single muscle fibers analyses that almost all fibers contained diminished cytochrome-c-oxidase activity. We will present in-situ hybridization showing that the focal ragged red appearance is associated with a high number of deleted mitochondrial DNA. A new family with the classical MELAS point mutation (mother and 3 sons) will be described. Detailed information of a MERRF patient without the classical mutation will be given.

This study was supported by the Deutsche Forschungsgemeinschaft and the Wilhelm Sander Stiftung.

51

NERVOUS SYSTEM INVOLVEMENT IN MITOCHONDRIAL MYOPATHIES WITH CHRONIC PROGRESSIVE EXTERNAL OPHTHALMOPLEGIA

Schubert M., Zierz S., Elek J. und Dengler R.

Neurologische Universitätsklinik Bonn, FRG

Mitochondrial myopathies with chronic progressive external ophthalmoplegia represent a distinct group among the mitochondrial myopathies. Apart from weakness of external eye muscles and other muscles clinical symptoms of different organ systems may occur. Some clinical and histopathological studies reported nervous system dysfunction. Only few electrophysiological investigations of central and peripheral nervous system involvement, however, are available. Therefore, we investigated 20 patients with mitochondrial myopathy with chronic progressive external ophthalmoplegia. Ages ranged from 14 to 69 years. Muscle biopsies revealed "ragged red fibres" and a focal cytochrome C oxidase deficiency in each patient. On clinical examination, involvement of the central nervous system was found in 4, of the peripheral nervous system in 1 and of both in 3 patients. Functions of the central and peripheral nervous system were assessed by means of nerve conduction studies and motor, somatosensory and auditory evoked potentials. Motor evoked potentials were carried out with a Magstim 200 magnetic stimulator. Results in patients were compared with normative values of our laboratory. Pathological results in electrophysiological tests pointing to involvement of the central nervous system only (motor, somatosensory and auditory evoked potentials) were found in 7 patients, of the peripheral nervous system only (nerve conduction studies, somatosensory and auditory evoked potentials) in 6 patients and of both in 6 patients. None of the patients with clinical signs of central or peripheral nervous system dysfunction showed overall normal findings on electrophysiological tests. Subclinical involvement of the central or peripheral nervous system was found in 11 patients. These studies may be useful as therapy control parameters.

52

TREATMENT OF OPHTALMOPLEGIA-PLUS WITH COENZYME Q

Petra Breul, Stephan Zierz und Felix Jerusalem
Neurologische Universitätsklinik Bonn

Twenty-six patients with mitochondrial encephalomyopathy presenting with progressive external ophthalmoplegia (CPEO) were treated with coenzyme Q_{10} (CoQ) for 12 months, 6 of them for more than 2 years. The daily dose of CoQ ranged from 33 to 150 mg corresponding to 0.6 to 2.6 mg/kg body weight. Serum lactate and pyruvate were measured at rest and during a standardized exercise test at 30 watt for 15 min. The maximal isometric muscle strength was assessed by quantitative tensiometry of 10 muscle groups. CoQ was measured in serum and muscle using an HPLC method. After one year of treatment CPEO had slightly improved in 4/26 patients. Intentional tremor and ataxia of gait had improved in 5/6 patients. Cardiac conduction defect, present in 9 patients and pigmentary retinopathy present in 15 patients did not improve. Muscle strength assessed by quantitative isometric tensiometry significantly increased after one year of treatment in 4/14 patients but deteriorated in 2 others. Treatment of 3 patients for 26-32 months resulted in no further improvement. Subjectively, 11/26 patients experienced improvement of endurance and exercise tolerance during therapy. These patients represented about 50% of the patients who had clear muscle weakness before treatment. Serum lactate at rest and during standardized exercise at 30 watt for 15 minutes decreased after one year of treatment by more than 25% in 10/24 patients but increased in 5 others. After one year of treatment the subgroup of patients with abnormally elevated serum lactate and elevated ratio of lactate/pyruvate at rest and during standardized exercise showed a significant reduction of lactate as well as of the ratio of lactate/pyruvate. There was no correlation between the increase of muscle strength and the decrease of lactate. There was also no correlation between the CoQ serum levels and the exercise induced rise of serum lactate before or during CoQ treatment. CoQ serum levels after 6 and 12 months of treatment showed significant correlations with the daily dose of CoQ per kg body weight. CoQ serum levels significantly increased during treatment after 6 months but decreased again after 12 months of treatment but still significantly higher than before treatment. After further treatment for 2 more years in 4 patients the CoQ serum levels remained unchanged. In 3 patients a second muscle biopsy could be obtained after one year of treatment. Although CoQ serum levels were clearly increased in these patients, there was no accumulation of CoQ in muscle. Two of these patients, however, showed a reduction of lactate at rest and during standardized exercise by more than 25% and muscle strength and ataxia had improved in one of these patients. The data indicate that CoQ therapy has only a marginal effect in only a few patients. There was no significant correlation between the reduction of pathologically elevated lactate and the improvement of clinical symptoms. There were no clear clinical or biochemical features common to those patients who clinically responded to CoQ therapy. The data do not exclude the possibility that higher CoQ doses might have a convincing beneficial effect on various symptoms of mitochondrial encephalomyopathies and especially on symptoms of the CNS.

53

Leber's Hereditary Optic Neuropathy: Mutations of the mitochondrial genome.

Seibel, P., Schneider, Ch., Lindner, A., Klopstock, Th., Toyka, K.-V. and Reichmann, H.

Neurologische Universitätsklinik
Josef-Schneider-Straße 11
D-8700 Würzburg

Leber's Hereditary Optic Neuropathy (LHON) is an inherited form of central optic nerve death associated with acute bilateral blindness. Cardiac dysrhythmia is also common and peripapillary microangiopathy is frequently seen in presymptomatic individuals. The age of onset ranges from adolescence to late adulthood (median age of onset is 20 to 24 years). The mode of inheritance of Leber's disease was originally regarded as an x-linked recessive disorder, but did not conform to mendelian principles. In contrast to x-linked inheritance, the descendants of affected males are never affected. This observation is compatible with the hypothesis that the disease is caused by variations of mitochondrial DNA, the only maternal inherited component of the human genome. Wallace (1) identified four mtDNA point-mutations that are sufficient in themselves to cause vision loss, and additional five mutations, which appear to contribute to LHON, though only in combination with other LHON mutations.

Results

We have analysed the mitochondrial genome of a patient with Leber's Hereditary Optic Neuropathy by restriction enzyme analysis and DNA sequencing. The most common of the mutations found by Wallace et al. (2) (G to A transition mutation at nucleotide pair 11778 of the human mitochondrial genome) was present in the mtDNA isolated from muscle tissue. The mutation at nt 11778 in the ND 4 gene of OXPHOS complex I (NADH-Dehydrogenase) converts the 340 th amino acid from an arginine to a histidine. The arginine is highly conserved between species during evolution, indicating functional importance. The mutation also removes a Sfa NI site on DNA level and thus enables us to identify the mutation easily by Sfa NI digestion of a PCR amplified fragment encompassing the mutation. The applied assay is easy to use in clinical diagnostics and can be scaled down to the non-invasive analysis of mtDNA obtained from plugged hairs of patients and relatives.

References:

1. Wallace DC (1992) Mitochondrial Genetics: A Paradigm for Aging and Degenerative Disease? Science 256:628-632.
2. Wallace DC, Singh G, Lott MT, Hodge JA, Schurr TG, Lezza AMS, Elsas LJ, Nikoskelainen EK (1988) Mitochondrial DNA Mutation Associated with Leber's Hereditary Optic Neuropathy. Science 242:1427-1430.

54

EYE MOVEMENT DISORDERS IN MYOTONIC DYSTROPHY

Hansen HC, Lueck CJ, Kennard C, Zangemeister WH
Dept. of Neurology, University Clinic Hamburg
Dept. of Neurology, The London Hospital London

In Dystrophia myotonica (DM) only occasional ocular motor findings have been reported and patients rarely complain about visuo-motor problems. This is surprising because the multisystem involvement known in this rather frequent myopathy of adulthood could lead to both peripheral and central eye movement disorders. Furthermore eye muscle involvement has been demonstrated histologically and the muscle membrane alteration presumably causing myotonia is expected to be generalized. Neuro-ophthalmological findings apart from the rather common cataract formation and ptosis are rare but include myotonic equivalents as tonic Bell's phenomenon and tonic convergence. Several authors reported of DM patients with progressive diplopia and a CPEO-like sydrome. While these reports would suggest deficits on a myopathic or myotonic basis, oculographic studies of smooth pursuit and saccades showed results that could be explained by central ocular motor involvement. The most consistent finding was reduced peak saccadic velocity leaving the question open at which level ocular motor function might be altered.

Different to previous studies the paradigm we used was predictive saccadic tracking with well-defined preceeding periods of ocular motor rest or activity in order to detect myotonic phenomena.

Saccades were elicited by a laser spot stimulus oscillating in a square wave manner between 10 degrees to left and right at different frequencies (0.5 and 1.0 Hz). With the head fixed tightly, we recorded eye movements with the infrared technique on audio-magnetic tape (bandwith DC to 150 Hz) and analyzed target position, amplitude and velocity off rectilinear UV-plotter charts. Saccadic amplitude and velocity data were collected 1) after preceeding resting periods of 1 minutes (eyes closed) and 2) going through 2 different frequencies up and down without resting interval. All seven patients studied were diagnosed of having DM with typical clinical and EMG myotonic findings and had unrestricted ocular movements in all directions. Ptosis was present in two patients and 5 age-matched hospital staff volunteers served as normal controls.

The course of predictive saccadic tracking was strikingly different in our DM patients with saccadic excursions that remained hypometric for the first 16 saccades on average. This reduced amplitude gain normalized gradually with a parallel increase of saccadic velocity. Peak saccadic velocities however never reached our control values (300 deg/sec compared to 421 deg/sec). A slightly more pronounced amplitude error was found in the higher frequency condition in contrast to our control data that did not show a similar effect. After antimyotonic treatment with tocainide the initial phase of saccadic amplitude build-up was markedly reduced or almost absent in two cases.

In our second series (4 untreated patients) we tested the effect of stimulus frequency to predictive saccades described elsewhere (Lueck et al. 1991). The expected increase of normalized velocities (i.e. peak sacc. velocity divided by natural logarithm of sacc. amplitude) was exaggerated in two patients, one of them nearly reaching near normal values.

Both experiments demonstrate the capability of the ocular motor system in patients with DM to improve performance with time (i.e. warm-up) resembling the well known myotonic phenomena present in these patients. The effects described here depend on well-defined experimental condition with respect to ocular motor activity before the testing session. This might help to explain why many studies only occasionally found reductions of peak saccadic velocity. These results contribute further evidence for a peripheral impairment as the cause of ocular slowing in DM patients.

55

MYOPATHY AND LIGNEOUS CONJUNCTIVITIS IN A CHILD

P. Krieg (1), W. Jost (1), J. Richter (1),
S. Loew (1), U. Mielke (2), KW. Ruprecht (3),
K. Remberger (4)

(1) Department of Paediatrics, University of the
Saarland, 6650 Homburg, Germany
(2) Department of Neurology, University of the
Saarland, 6650 Homburg, Germany
(3) Department of Ophthalmology, University of the
Saarland, 6650 Homburg, Germany
(4) Department of Pathology, University of the
Saarland, 6650 Homburg, Germany

A term girl presents at the age of 6 months with muscular hypotonia and a delay in attaining developmental milestones. At the age of 8 months two generalized seizures were noted. 9 months later severe myoclonic-astatic seizures occurred. By the age of 22 months the child developed a pseudomembranous conjunctivitis with thickening of the upper eyelid and moderate amount of discharge. First only the right eye was affected, later both eyes were involved. The girl was treated with different therapies including topical steroids, local cyclosporin A, and alpha-chymotrypsin without discernible improvement. The large membranes were removed surgically on two occassions, but they recurred immediately. Histologically the diagnosis of ligneous conjunctivitis was made. Eosinophilic hyaline material, areas of granulation tissue, and areas of cellular infiltrations were seen. The components of the infiltrations included lymphocytes (T- and B-cells) and CD-38 positive macrophages. Immunoglobulins were found in the hyaline material.

The now 3-year-old girl still shows a delay in her development especially in speech production and in motor milestones, but a deterioration is not evident. Of note in her appearance is - besides her eye problems - a muscle hypotrophy. The child is treated with anticonvulsants and physical therapy. The diagnostic procedures did not imply any neurologic metabolic disorder especially any storage disease. Only a permanent raise of the serum creatine kinase was seen. The muscle biopsy revealed signs of a primary vasculitic process with consecutive muscle fiber degeneration.

Ligneous conjunctivitis is a rare form of chronic membranous conjunctivitis with beginning usually in the childhood. The disease is often refractory to therapy and has a marked tendency to recurrences. The pathogenesis is not known. Numerous causes have been proposed. The combination of ligneous conjunctivitis and a muscular process has not been described so far. In the present case a myopathy probably due to primary vasculitis occurred together with the eye symptoms. This supports the hypothesis of an underlying systemic immune disorder in ligneous conjunctivitis. If there exists an association with the seizures and the delay of development, remains unknown.

Platform session II
Therapy monitoring

56

Effect of different hemisphere-specific brain activities on hemodynamics in the middle cerebral artery territory

G. Matzander, J. Klingelhöfer, I. Wittich, D. Sander, B. Conrad

Department of Neurology, Technical University of Munich, Möhlstraße 28, W-8000 München 80

Different brain activities cause specific patterns of cerebral activation in the two hemispheres which may result in regional differences in cerebral blood flow. In the present study, we evaluated the rapid alterations in cerebral perfusion in both middle cerebral arteries during different hemispheric-specific brain activities and established the dynamics of these changes.

The flow velocity changes of the right and left middle cerebral artery were investigated in 16 right-handed healthy subjects using pulsed Doppler systems (2 MHz) unilaterally or bilaterally simultaneously during hemisphere-specific brain activities in the form 1) of spatial tasks (comparison of wooden figures presented visually and for tactile sensation by the right and the left hand respectively), 2) pure finger activities (right and left hand), 3) a memory task (memorization and recall of picture material) and 4) acustic stimuli (white noise, speech, music). In some subjects, the endexpiratory CO_2 content and peripheral arterial blood pressure were registered simultaneously.

Significant increases of the flow velocities up to 9% averaged over several investigations could be detected ith all stimulation tasks compared to the resting phases. In the hemisphere contralateral to the executing hand, significantly higher flow velocity increases were shown than in the ipsilateral hemisphere in performance of visual motor-spatial tasks and finger activities. In addition, there were greater flow velocity increases in the right middle cerebral artery than in the left middle cerebral artery in the performance of spatial tasks although not in the pure finger activities. Side differences in the reactive flow velocity increases were also found in performance of the memory test (right > left). Presentation of white noise led to small velocity increases which were equal in the two middle cerebral arteries, whereas significantly higher increases were measured with speech in the left and with music in the right middle cerebral artery. The time course of the flow velocity reaction showed a rapid initial rise with an initial maximum after 4s to 5 s and steady-state phases after a further 5s to 15s.

The flow velocity alterations during functional brain activation are consistent with the results of cerebral blood flow measurements. The side differences conform to concepts on the functional anatomy of the cortex. The rather uniform flow velocity reactions at the beginning of the activation phases indicate that the development of specific cortical activation patterns is initially preceded by a non-specific cortical reaction. The time course of the flow velocity reactions is similar to that measured in the posterior cerebral artery in visual stimulation and reflects the vascular reaction observed in sensory stimulation in animal experiments.

57

Doppler-CO$_2$-Test in Patients with Vertebrobasilar Ischemia

Ch.Kessler, M.v.Maravic, M.Müller, D.Dorndorf, and D.Kömpf

Department of Neurology, Medizinische Universität zu Lübeck, Lübeck, F.R.G.

Prognostic factors which influence the outcome of patients with vertebrobasilar ischemia (VBI) are still unknown. In order to evaluate the role of an impaired vasomotor reactivity (VMR) in the basilar artery for the prognosis of VBI-patients we conducted a prospective study in 56 patients (38m, 18f, mean age 62.3. +13.4y). 14 patients suffered from a brainstem TIA, 34 patients had a completed brainstem stroke and 8 patients an infarction in the area of the posterior cerebral artery (PCA). The mean follow-up time was 12.6 +3,1 month. During the follow-up a neurological examination including the assessment of the Barthel-index of daily life activity as well as a special designed VBI-score were performed at the acute state and at tree month intervals. The follow-up examinations included an cw-Doppler sonography of the extracranial arteries and the Doppler-CO$_2$-Test in the basilar artery. Using a transcranial Doppler device with a 2 mHz probe we insonated the basilar artery via the transnuchal window in a depth between 9 and 11 cm. First the baseline mean flow velocities were measured than the patients were asked to inhale increasing concentrations of CO$_2$ up to an endtidal CO$_2$-concentration of 8.5 Vol%. During this procedure the procental increase of basilar blood flow velocities was calculaed contineously.

As a result, we found a significant reduction of the procental dilatation reserve (%DR) in patients with brainstem-TIA (39.4 +8.3 %) and completed brainstem stroke (32.6 +9.9) as compared to normal controls (53.0 +9.2) and patients with PCA infarctions (52 +12.6; $p < 0.05$). During the follow up-period both the Barthel-index as well as the VBI-score improved significantly ($p < 0.05$) patients with brainstem TIA and brainstem Stroke, but not in patients with PCA infarctions. In 13 patients with an profoundly decreased %DR under 30%, the %DR remained low and the clinical VBI-score did not improved substantially during the follow up period. Our findings show that the Doppler-CO$_2$-Test in the basilar artery may be useful to estimate the prognosis of patients with VBI.

58

Diagnostic Accuracy of Ultrasound Methods in the Evaluation of Vertebral Arteries

Delcker A, Timmann D, Diener HC,
Department of Neurology, University of Essen, FRG

Duplex sonography and color coded duplex sonography (CCDS) have improved the evaluation of the hemodynamic situation in the vertebral arteries (VA). A reliable differentiation between a normal vessel, hypoplasia, stenosis and occlusion of VA is possible by CCDS. Color flow systems make it easy to place the Doppler sample volume within the colored vertebral artery and to evaluate the Doppler angle (between 45° to 60°) for reliable measurements of velocity spectra. This possibility does not exist in continuous-wave Doppler sonography (CWD) or transcranial Doppler sonography (TCD).

In a prospective study, 359 unselected patients (148 females, 211 males, AM +- SD: 55 +- 18 years) were examined with CCDS, CWD and TCD in a 4-month period. For evaluation of CWD and TCD Doppler findings we employed the criteria described by Büdingen (CWD; 1) and by Aaslid (TCD; 2). CCDS was used as the reference method (3). CCDS showed abnormalities in 4.4% (n=32) of VA (hypoplasia < 2 mm: 1.9%; stenosis: 1.7%; occlusion: 0.8 %). CWD had a sensitivity of 100% and a specificity of 27% for the detection of unusual vertebral arteries. For TCD these values were 38% and 58% respectively. TCD was unable to differentiate between hypoplasia, proximal stenosis and a VA of normal size.

Our study showed that CW - Doppler is a useful screening examination to find pathological findings of vertebral arteries. In cases of abnormalities in CW - Doppler a color coded duplex sonography should be added.

References:

(1) Büdingen HJ, Von Reutern GM, Freund HJ (1976) The selective examination of the neck arteries by directional Doppler sonography. Arch Psychiatr Nervenkr 222:177-190

(2) Aaslid R, Markwalder TM, Nornes H (1982) Noninvasive transcranial Doppler ultrasound recording of flow velocity in basal cerebral arteries. J Neurosurg 57:769-774

(3) Delcker A, Diener HC (1992) Color coded duplex sonography in the evaluation of vertebral arteries. Imaging 59:16-21

59

COLOR DOPPLER IMAGING IN PATIENTS WITH DISSECTIONS OF THE EXTRACRANIAL ARTERIES

M.Kaps, S.Trittmacher, G.Seidel, M.S.Damian
Neurologische Klinik und Neuroradiologie der Justus-Liebig-Universität, D-6300 Giessen, FRG.

Background: The ultrasonic findings in arterial dissections are as varied as their morphological features. Intimal flaps and "double lumen" can be considered specific, but further abnormalities reported in the literature are also observed in other vascular diseases. Ultrasonic techniques are now recognized as the primary modality for early diagnosis [1] [2] [4]. We investigated the potential of Color Doppler Imaging (**CDI**) in this context.

Method: CDI follow up examinations were performed in 7 patients with arterial dissections confirmed by angiography. Extracranial sonography was done using 7.5 MHz linear and 5 MHz sector probes, and transcranial studies using a 2.5 MHz sector transducer (Sonos 1000 Hewlett Packard).

Results: The Internal Carotid Artery (**ICA**) was the site of dissection in 6 cases and the Vertebral Artery (**VA**) in one case. Angiography revealed fibromuscular dysplasia in one patient, 3 patients had a history of trauma, 4 cases were spontaneous. Tapered occlusions of the ICA were demonstrated by Duplex sonography in 5 cases; one of these later recanalized. A membrane crossing the ICA lumen was seen in one case. A traumatic pseudoaneurysm near the base of the skull was identified by color coding in a patient with a fracture of the posterior arch of the second cervical vertebra. In a further case a "string sign", indicating a long stenosis of the V1 segment of the VA, could only be visualized by Duplex sonography subsequently to CDI identification of pathology.

Transcranial Color Doppler Imaging (**TCDI**) was performed in 6 patients. A significant and clinically relevant reduction of ipsilateral Middle Cerebral Artery perfusion was only observed in one case of ICA occlusion (> 30% side difference of maximum systolic velocity).

Conclusion: Efficiency in diagnosing dissections is enhanced by simultaneous imaging of structural and functional findings. Color Coding enables better identification of residual lumen than conventional ultrasound. Pathological flow in aneurysmatic structures can be demonstrated under favourable conditions. Abnormalities near the base of the skull, which pose problems for Duplex sonography, are visualized satisfactorily. VA pathology in the region of the aortic arch is also more readily detected, as orthograde insonation angles create difficulties in B-mode but facilitate CDI. Unequivocal identification of basal cerebral arteries by TCDI allows better evaluation of intracranial hemodynamics than previously possible. The results with this new technique are otherwise comparable to findings earlier made with conventional transcranial Doppler sonography [3].

References

1. De Bray JM, Dubas F, Joseph PA, Causeret H, Pasquier JP, Emile E (1989) Etude ultrasonique de 22 dissections carotidiennes. Rev Neurol 145: 702-709.
2. Hennerici M, Steinke W, Rautenberg W (1989) High-resistance Doppler flow pattern in extracranial carotid dissection. Arch Neurol 46:670-672.
3. Kaps M, Dorndorf W, Damian MS, Agnoli L (1990) Intracranial haemodynamics in patients with spontaneous carotid dissection. Eur Arch Psychiatr Neurol Sci 239:246-256.
4. Sturzenegger M (1991) Ultrasound findings in spontaneous carotid artery dissection. Arch Neurol 48: 1057-1063.

60

TCD-MONITORING OF THERAPEUTIC CAROTID OCCLUSIONS

A. Thie, M. Carvajal-Lizano, J. Steinmetz, F. Zanella*, K. Spitzer, H. Zeumer*
Neurologische Klinik und Abt. f. Neuroradiologie*
Universitäts-Krankenhaus Eppendorf, Hamburg

Background and objectives:
Percutaneous transarterial therapeutic occlusion of the internal carotid artery (ICA) bears the risk of cerebral ischemia in the distal vascular territories due to insufficient collateral channels. We assessed the value of hemodynamic monitoring with transcranial Doppler ultrasound (TCD) during this intervention, and to establish criteria of imminent hemodynamic compromise.

Patients and methods:
We studied 12 consecutive patients who underwent ICA occlusion for therapy of giant aneurysms (n=5), arteriovenous fistulae (n=2) or tumors (n=5). Mean blood flow velocities (MBFV) and pulsatility indices (PI) were continuously measured in the ipsilateral middle cerebral artery (MCA) with a fixed 2-MHz probe. In 8 patients, changes of MBFV to motor stimulation (intermittent fist clenching and sequential finger movements) were recorded before and after ICA occlusion to test vasoreactivity.

Results:
Two patients suffered transient ischemic symptoms shortly after ICA occlusion due to hemodynamic compromise. In these patients, MBFV in the MCA dropped to values below 50% of those before occlusion. In the asymptomatic patients, MBFV were reduced by a mean of 20% (range, 0-31%). The decrease of PI was higher in symptomatic (mean, 38%) than in asymptomatic patients (mean, 21%), but varied widely (range, 0-49%). Motor vaso-reactivity after occlusion showed major individual differences in this sample, but was markedly reduced or abolished in symptomatic patients. In 2 asymptomatic patients, MBFV in the MCA were completely suppressed immediately after occlusion, but increased continuously over several minutes to levels before occlusion.

Conclusions:
Drop of MBFV in the MCA by 50% or more with concomitant marked decrease of PI and reduction of motor vasoreactivity may herald risk of ischemic damage in patients undergoing therapeutic ICA occlusion. We recommend the use of TCD monitoring during this intervention to rapidly detect insufficiency of collateral channels.

61

DOPPLER ULTRASOUND STUDIES AFTER PERCUTANEOUS TRANSLUMINAL ANGIOPLASTY OF BRAIN-SUPPLYING ARTERIES

J. Steinmetz, A. Thie, F. Zanella, K. Kunze, H. Zeumer

Neurologische Universitätsklinik Hamburg-Eppendorf

Percutaneous transluminal angioplasty (PTA) is a treatment option for selected stenoses of the brain-supplying arteries. Long-term clinical results and restenosis rates remain to be fully evaluated.

We studied 36 patients (24 men, 12 women) with extracranial and transcranial Doppler ultrasound before, shortly after and during follow-up 6 and 12 months (maximum, 4 years) after PTA. Vascular lesions included high-grade stenosis at the origin of the internal carotid (n=7) or vertebral artery (n=7), the proximal subclavian artery (n=18) and the innominate artery (n=4).

Shortly after PTA, the grade of stenosis was significantly reduced in 94% of lesions (n=34) according the hemodynamic criteria. In subclavian stenosis, 15 patients (83%) exhibited latent or overt steal phenomena before PTA that were still present, but attenuated in 8 patients (44%) after PTA. Marked improvement of hemodynamic compromise or steal phenomena was detected in all patients with innominate artery lesions after PTA. All patients with carotid stenosis showed a good hemodynamic response to treatment with reversal of collateral pathways (in 5 of 5 patients). PTA resulted in marked reduction of stenosis in 5 of 7 vertebral lesions. During follow-up, this favorable hemodynamic response to treatment was maintained on ultrasonic examination. We found no evidence of restenosis in any patient.

Doppler ultrasound is a feasible method to document early and long-term hemodynamic results after PTA.

62

Preoperative Stroke Risk Assessment is Improved by a Multimodal Carotid Balloon Occlusion Test

[1]Ries F., [2]Keller E., [3]Grünwald F., [1]Honisch C., [4]Rosanowski F., [5]Kurthen M., [2]Solymosi L.
Departments of [1]Neurology, [2]Neuroradiology, [3]Nuclear Medicine, [4]ENT Clinic, [5]Neurosurgery, University Hospital Bonn, FRG

Iatrogenic occlusion of the common or internal carotid artery may be inevitable for therapeutical reasons, i.e. in most radical surgery of head and neck tumors or in case of giant carotid aneurysms to be occluded by balloon embolisation. The inherent stroke risk is evident. A multimodal preoperative risk assessment by carotid balloon occlusion test including brain perfusion measurement and EEG monitoring at rest and under occlusion was completed by a concomitant test of the cerebrovascular reserve capacity (CVRC) under carotid occlusion, as measured by transcranial Doppler sonography. This procedure should allow to delineate patients at high risk for postoperative ischemic infarction.

Methods and Patients Collective
A total of 38 patients (26 male, 12 female, mean age 63.5 years, range 22-86 years), with head and neck tumors (n=32) and giant internal carotid aneurysms (n=6) was investigated.
The perocclusive test battery included neurological examination, continuous monitoring by ECG, blood pressure, EEG and, in the last 10 patients, 2 MHz transcranial Doppler investigation of the MCA.
After catheterization of the internal carotid artery in local anesthesia, balloon inflation was maintained for 10 minutes. Prolonged hemispheric EEG alterations, a neurological deficit mentioned spontaneously by the patient or manifest in the repeated neurological examination were considered pathologic.
The radioactive tracer (^{99}Tc-HMPAO) was injected i.v. 30 seconds following the onset of carotid occlusion. In case of pathological SPECT findings, a baseline SPECT was performed before surgery.

Results
Balloon occlusion had to be interrupted in 8 patients due to a relevant delta focus in EEG monitoring without neurological abnormalities (n=4) respectively with neurological deficits (n=4), additionally corresponding in 3/4 patients to pathological SPECT findings. An intraoperative occlusion was not recommended in this group.
In 30 patients, there were no EEG or neurological abnormalities. One patient with a normal SPECT as well was occluded without complications. An asymmetrical hemispheric perfusion was found in 17/30 patients. Out of 7/17 patients with moderate SPECT asymmetry, 3 were occluded without neurological complications. In 10/17 patients with a severe hypoperfusion, 4 patients had to be occluded, and 3/4 suffered neurological deficits.
In order to quantify this preoperative risk evaluation, an enlarged test battery additionally included continuous transcranial Doppler monitoring before occlusion, during a short test occlusion at rest (for 2') and following injection of 1g acetazolamide for assessing CVRC under occlusion conditions.
Preliminary results in 10/38 patients (6 male, 4 female, mean age 56.7 yrs., range 22-86 yrs.) allow a continuous evaluation of direct hemodynamic effects of balloon occlusion in different phases of both the test occlusion at rest and during the 10' occlusion with CVR assessment, including the effect of collateral pathways. Furthermore, assessment of the CVRC under occlusion simulates changing perfusion requirements which may occur postoperatively.

Summary
intraoperative occlusion was considered prospective low risk in 13/30 patients. A permanent occlusion was performed in 8/30 cases. In 5/8 patients, there was no postocclusive deficit, even in presence of a severe SPECT asymmetry under occlusion in 1 patient. In 3/8 definitely occluded patients, one suffered a small embolic infarction (related to the rupture of a detached balloon in a giant aneurysm). In 2/8 patients with a subsequent hemodynamic ischemic infarction, preoperative EEG monitoring and neurological testing were normal in presence of pathological SPECT findings.
The combined multimodal evaluation of cortical function, brain perfusion and hemodynamics at rest as well as under occlusion without and with CVR measurement should allow a highly reliable preoperative risk assessment in case of permanent carotid occlusion.

63

EXAMPLES OF FUNCTIONAL REORGANISATION OF THE HUMAN CEREBRAL CORTEX AFTER CAPSULAR INFARCTS - A PET-ACTIVATION STUDY

CORNELIUS WEILLER, KARL J FRISTON, RICHARD SJ FRACKOWIAK

Neurologische Klinik Essen FRG; Hammersmith Hospital, London, UK

Recovery of function after stroke is often observed, although the morphological lesion that originally caused the deficit persists. In a previous study on a group of patients in recovery from motor stroke due to a striatocapsular infarct we found a bilateral activation of motorsystems and recruitment of additional brain regions, functionally connected with the motor system. We have now developed a technique to assess changes in regional cerebral blood flow (rCBF) during a sequential finger oppostion task with positron emission tomographie in individual patients.

The pattern of cortical activation was compared individually in eight patients with a capsular infarct with 10 normal controls. The paradigm was sequential finger to thumb opposition, a function that originally was paralyzed in the patients. Despite disruption of the pyramidal tract in the internal capsule complete recovery of function had occurred. After stereotactic transformation and normalisation for global flow differences, comparisons were done on a pixel by pixel basis.

As in our group study, we found an above normal rCBF increase during the task in almost all patients bilaterally in the insula and the parietal cortex (area 40) and in the ipsilateral premotor cortex, basal ganglia and contralateral cerebellum. In addition there was an activation of the supplemantary motor cortex in most patients.
In only four patients an additional activation in the contralateral sensorimotor cortex was found along it's ventral extent, more than a centimeter more caudally as the area activated by finger opposition in normals. This region of the primary sensorimotor cortex is normally thought of having outputs to the face. All four patients had a posterior lesion affecting the posterior part of the posterior limb of the internal capsule, sparing the anterior llimb, the genu and the anterior part of the posterior limb. No extension of the sensorimotor cortex was found in patients wiht anterior lesions.

The ipsilateral primary sensorimotor cortex was activated in only four patients, all of whom exhibited associated movements of the primarily unaffected hand when attempting to move the previously plegic hand.

There is considerable scope for functional plasticity within the adult human motor cortex. Complete recovery from capsular motor stroke is associated with individually different patterns of functional reorganisation. Because of the somatotopic organisation of the pyramidal tract, the site of a subcortical lesion detemermines the pattern of reorganisation in the cerebral cortex.

64

IN VIVO 1H-NMR SPECTROSCOPY (MRS) OF THE BRAIN AFTER TEMPORARY ISCHEMIA

L. Harms, S. Enchtuja, G. Timm, R. Zschenderlein, B. Schnackenburg, S. Walter

Dept. of Neurology, Dept. of Diagnostic Radiology, Humboldt-University, Charité, Berlin

Introduction: 1H-nuclear magnetic resonance spectroscopy is a method to monitor in vivo the concentrations of metabolites in the brain, such as N-Acetyl-aspartate (NAA), phosphocholine (Pch), lactate (Lac) and phosphocreatine (Pcr). Better understanding of the tissue metabolism will have implications for treatment. Under normal conditions brain tissue derives its energy through oxidative metabolism. Under anaerobic conditions lactate is produced. Animal studies and studies in completed stroke in humans have demonstrated that ischemia leads to increased lactate concentration and decreased energy-rich phosphates and tissue pH. The influence of subclinically reduced cerebral blood flow on this metabolism is not clear. It is possible to investigate a well defined volume of the human brain in the region of estimated decreased perfusion. Water-suppressed localized proton magnetic resonance spectroscopy was performed with the goal to estimate brain lactate and NAA after transient ischemic attacks (TIA) and reversible ischemic neurological deficit (RIND) in order to prove the hypothesis that reduction of cerebral blood flow without clinical signs is associated with increased concentration of lactate.

Methods: Spectroscopic results of 15 patients with ischemic disturbances were compared with data of 10 healthy volunteers. Seven of the patients had TIAs (group 1), eight of them had RINDs (group 2). All were examined in the region of reduced cerebral blood flow and in the contralateral area of the brain at least six weeks after the last clinical symptom. The reduction of cerebral blood flow was estimated with the help of the results of ultrasound-Doppler and/or Xenon-CT. No morphological defects could be detected by CT or NMR. In vivo 1H-MRS was performed with water suppression by selective inversion pulses using 1.5 T (Gyroscan S15, Philips). The volume of interest (20x20x40 mm) was localized in transversal images. The spectra were obtained using the following parameters: TR = 2 sec, TE = 272 msec, sample frequency 1kHz, 1024 samples, 256 measurements. In the standard processing of spectra zero filling 4 K, Fourier transformation and phase correction were used. Evaluation of ratio PCh to PCr, NAA to PCh and NAA to lactate was used to describe metabolic changes mathematically.

Results: No changes of PCh/PCr and NAA/PCr ratios could be found in the three groups. In 12 patients lactate in different concentrations was detected. Some of the patients with RINDs had considerable differences between pathological area and contralateral hemisphere. There was no strong correlation between increased concentration of lactate and the degree of stenosis or measured reduction of cerebral blood flow.

Discussion: The results suggest that also subclinical reduction of the cerebral blood flow can provide an increased concentration of lactate in the brain. The clinical importance of these preliminary findings is unclear. Its possible that it is a compensation or a serious sign making the treatment of the underlying stenosis urgently necessary. We speculate that lactate in this relation may be a marker of reversible brain disturbances or reduced cerebral blood flow. It seems that proton MRS is a sensitive indicator of ischemia. Further studies which investigate the same patients pre-and postoperative should provide a better understanding of the phenomenon.

References:
1. Berkelbach van der Sprenkel JW, Luyten PR, van Rijen PC, Tulleken CAF, den Hollander JA (1988) Cerebral Lactate detected by regional proton magnetic resonance spectroscopy in a patient with cerebral infarction. Stroke 1: 73-792
2. Hossmann KA (1991) Untersuchungen der experimentellen zerebralen Ischämie mit NMR-Spektroskopie. Drug Res. 41: 292-297
3. Kucharczyk J, Moseley M, Kurhanewicz J, Norman D (1989) MRS of ischemic/hypoxic brain disease. Investigative Radiology 24: 951-954
4. Peeling J, Wong D, Sutherland GR (1989) Nuclear magnetic resonance study of regional metabolism after forebrain ischemia in rats. Stroke 5: 633-640
5. Rosenberg GA, White J, Gasparovic C, Crisostomo EA, Griffey RH ((1991) Effect of hypoxia on cerebral metabolites measured by proton nuclear magnetic resonance spectroscopy in rats. Stroke 1:73-79

65

Classification of rating-scale-data using an artificial neural net

P.H.Kraus[1], T.Fritsch[2], P.Tran-Gia[2], H.Przuntek[3]

[1] Univ.of Würzburg, Dept.of Psychiatry, [2] Univ.of Würzburg, Dept.of Computer Science, [3] Univ.of Bochum, Dept.of Neurology

The over-all-score of an assessment of clinical stages with help of rating scales is problematic: Because of the unknown weights of the items and the nonlinearity of the interrelation between real expression of the symptoms and rated values the correlation between sum-scores and an integrative assessment by an expert is only low.

In the present examination data of 666 de-novo Parkinsonian patients of a multicenter study were analysed concerning the question how different scores reflect the same clinical state.

All 10 items of the Webster rating scale (which possesses 4 stages for each item) and the rating following Hoehn and Yahr (which is more integrative and puts main emphasis of different symptoms) were analysed with multivariate linear statistical methods (multiple regression and discriminant analysis) in an explorative way.

It should be estimated, to what degree the results of both scales represent the same information.

Both proceedings yielded linear models which were used for a kind of 'prediction' for the same data set: It was used to recognize the Hoehn and Yahr staging out of the staging with the Webster rating scale.

Since the patients only showed low symptoms we only found Hoehn and Yahr stages from 1 to 4 (129 patients stage 1, 265 patients stage 2, 231 patients stage 3 and 41 patients stage 4).

Multiple regression as well as discriminant analysis yielded a quote of right classification of about 50 %. The discriminant analysis was superior to the multiple regression for extreme ratings (Hoehn and Yahr stage 1 and 4).

To make a comparison: The value of right classification by a random selection is 25 % for the 4 stages of the Hoehn and Yahr scale.

For the same classification an artificial neural net of Kohonen type was used, which interprets the data as input vectors and extracts features following predefined criteria for similarity. The net learned competitively the probability density function of the input vectors and adapted in a self-organizing way the weights interconnecting the input neurons with the neurons of the two-dimensional mapping area. The centroids of the vector clusters were mapped to the best-matching neurons. The used algorithm is able to build clusters by use of a modified processing which can be assigned to the learning vector quantization method (Linde, Buzo, Gray).

Since the net is adaptive, the input space can be expanded with the same quality of recognition.

For a net of 40 to 40 neurons we yielded a nonlinear right classification of about 90 % for the 4 stages of Hoehn and Yahr.

The 10 % of patients which were not classified correctly can be interpreted as outliers.

It is visible that the classification model of the neural net is superior to that of (inappropriate) linear statistical methods.

The usefulnes for classification of external data which were not learned by the net has still to be examined.

For practice a similar proceeding with an integrative expert rating as 'predictor' can yield a more intelligent alternative to the assessment of sum-scores.

66

PROGNET - Prognostic Neuronal Network in neurology.

Klaus Spitzer, Klaus Kunze, Andreas Thie
Neurologische Universitätsklinik Hamburg-Eppendorf

It is important to recognize in good time trends in the number of beds occupled, duration of hospitalization and incidence of neurological diseases treated in hospital in order to attain optimal utilization of staff and equipment capacities of a neurological hospital. The Prognostic Neuronal Network (PROGNET) was developed to predict these parameters. An artificial neuronal network is a computer program generating a model of a group of interacting natural neurons and simulating human problem-solving strategies by parallel information processing. PROGNET evaluates the information contained in the data bank of the Neurology Division at the University of Hamburg. This data bank has stored the administrative data, diagnoses and concomitant diseases of about 10,000 inpatients treated at the hospital during the last seven years. The prototype provides the following prognoses for the period of one week and one month: expected bed utilization, duration of hospital treatment, age and sex distribution, number of admissions with individual diagnoses, incidence of concomitant diseases and complications, number of deaths, number of transfers. The predictions of the neuronal network have a precision of about 70%.

67

ANTICOAGULATION VERSUS ACETYL SALICYLIC ACID IN CAROTID DISSECTION

G.Krämer for the German Carotid Artery Dissection (GECAD) Study Group
Department of Neurology, University Hospital of Mainz

In the literature, data exist describing a favourable prognosis of extracranial internal carotid artery dissection (ICAD) with almost complete recovery of clinical symptoms and signs in at least 80% of patients (Hart and Easton 1985). In contrast, other authors refer to a mortality rate of 25% of patients within the acute phase and a disabling neurological deficit in about 30-40% of the survivors (e.g. Bogousslavsky et al 1987).

The therapy of extracranial ICAD is ill defined and controversial with widespread use of potentially harmful anticoagulation in most centres and use of acetyl salicylic acid (ASS) only in others. In view of the great variability in clinical manifestation and prognosis of the disease, up to now therapeutic decisions are based on empirical data and theroretical considerations. The value and the risk-benefit-ratio of anticoagulants in the treatment of ICAD is still unclear. So far, there are no data from controlled clinical studies.

Therefore, 10 departments of Neurology in Germany developed a study protocol comparing two therapeutic strategies in a prospective and randomized trial:
- anticoagulation (heparin initially, oral anticoagulants later) in the acute phase followed by ASS, versus
- ASS only for the complete treatment period.

Unilateral ICAD has to be confirmed angiographically, and focal non-neurological or neurological signs and symptoms (ipsilateral pain in the neck or periorbital region, Horner's syndrome, pulsatile tinnitus or lesions of the lower cranial nerves) or signs of retinal or cerebral ischemia (transient or permanent) have to be present.

Anticoagulation consists of heparin (bolus of 5.000 I.U. initially and 1.000 i.U. per hour thereafter adjusted as necessary to achieve an INR value between 1.5 and 2.7) for 2-6 weeks followed by phenprocoumon (Marcumar,) until the end of the third month after the initial event. The ASS dosis is 250-300 mg per day which can be decreased to 100 mg in the presence of gastrointestinal side effects.
The criteria for therapeutic efficacy are primary prevention (retinal and cerebral infarcts or death) as well as secondary prevention. The follow-up period is one year.

With the assumption of a possible decrease of the combined event rate for primary target criteria of 50%, an alpha-error of 0.05 and a power of 0.8, about 200 patients have to be included in the study. With more than 25 participating centers and estimated 3 patients per hospital per year a recruitment period of 3 years has to be expected. The trial has started already, but interested centres can still participate.

References:
Bogousslavsky J, Despland PA, Regli F (1987) Spontaneuos carotid dissection with acute stroke. Arch Neurol 44: 134-137
Hart RG, Easton JD (1985) Dissections. Stroke 16: 925-927

68

Design of a double-blind cross-over study for the evaluation of the pharmacologic effects of a xanthin-derivative on patients with progressive muscular dystrophy.

R. Lindemuth, U. Mielke, W. Jost, I. Maurer, A. Marian, W. Kuhn*.
Universitätsnervenklinik-Neurologie
D-6650 Homburg/Saar
*Fraunhofer-Institut Abt. Medizintechnik
D-6670 St. Ingbert

A causal medicamental therapy for the progressive muscular dystrophies is not available up to now. Possible targets of a phamacological intervention are the enhancement of the contraction force, the performance, and the resistance to fatigue of the muscle, an increase of the muscular perfusion , a better utilisation of oxygen and changes in the lactate level. Beside that one has to take into consideration the different effects on the aerobic and anaerobic metabolism.
In animal experiments with a xanthin-derivative it has been shown a positive effect on the running performance, the muscle contraction force and the fatigue of muscles with limited blood supply. The recovering time for the PCr/Pi-level was ameliorated. Both on hypoxic and on control muscle the xanthin-derivative reduced the fraction of glycolytic fibres and changed the lactate dehydrogenase-activities. Possible effects of this derivative are the amelioration of the substrate supply of the muscle fibre or effects on the muscle energy metabolism, e. g. through the known effects of the methylxanthines on the cyclic nucleotide phosphodiesterase or the adenosine receptors.
It will be presented the results of a recently finished double-blinded cross-over pilot study with this agent. Course parameters are the clinical muscle score (MRC) and a standardized performance test: on the basis of bicycle ergometry heart-rate, ventilation, oxygen consumption, and oxygen-pulse are continuously monitored. The blood values for lactate, pyruvate, and ammonia are determined at rest, at peak performance, and during the recovery period. 31-P-NMR spectroscopy was performed on the m. vastus medialis using a 1.5 Tesla magnetic coil. The spectra were obtained at rest, during standardized ergometric exercise and the recovery period.
The preliminary results of the study suggest that the standardized test protocol applied in the presented study is valid for the evaluation of pharmacological effects on skeletal muscle - muscular dystrophy.

69

Value of Coma Scales for the early evaluation of prognosis in primarily comatose patients

M.J.Hilz, U.Faatz, M.Weis,.F.Erbguth, B.Neundörfer

It would be desirable to be able to establish an early evaluation of outcome and prognosis even in primarily comatose patients. We investigated 7 different coma scales and tried to find out wether prognostic estimations are possible in early stages of disease.

Methods: In our study we included only patients who were already comatose on admission. We examined 75 patients (35 men/40 women, age 20 to 87 yrs., mean 64.1 yrs., SD 15.5) admitted on our neurological ICU on the day of admission, as well as on the next 4 days. 26 patients had intra-cerebral haematomas, 24 cerebral-and 10 brainstem infarcts, 9 encephalitis, 6 had other diseases. We graded these patients according to 3 clinical scales (Grading after Gerstenbrand and Lücking, Grading after Bozza-Marrubini and after Frowein) and 4 scoring systems (Glasgow Coma Scale, Innsbruck Coma Scale (ICS), Munich Coma Scale, Erlanger Funktions-psychose Skala B (FPSB)). After 10 month the outcome of the patients was classified into the Glasgow Outcome Scale (GOS). For the statistical correlation we used the Pearson Correlation.

Results: On reviewing the outcome, 57.5% were dead, o% apallic, 25.9% were severely and 9.6% were moderately disabled, 4% were in a good condition. As the correlation coefficients (r) showed, non of the gradings correlated with outcome on the day of admission. On the first day after admission the only score system which correlated with the GOS was the ICS (r=0.32, p<0.01), out of the clinical gradings the classification according to Bozza-Marrubini (r=0.27, p<0.05) and to Gerstenbrand and Lücking (r=0.28, p<0.05). On the following days of illness the GOS always correlated significantly with all 7 scales. The Frowein Scale and the FPSB correlated only minimally with the GOS. The ICS gave the earliest and best overall correlation with the GOS.

Discussion: Our investigations showed that only the ICS made it possible for one to make a relatively accurate evaluation of the outcome in early stages of disease, in fact as early as from the first day following admission. This early correlation with outcome may probably be due to the fact that the ICS, out of the gradings tested, correlates best with the clinical findings (1,2). We have obtained similar results in earlier studies which showed that the ICS is considerably appropriate for assessing the course of patients with reduced level of conscious-ness and those in coma (2). The other scores only correlate later on, that is to say on the following days of examination, with the GOS. Furthermore the FPSB and the Frowein Scale showed the worst correlation with outcome. This is due to the fact that out of the 33 items evaluated with the FPSB only 6 are neurological signs; although the Frowein Scale allows for fast and adequate evaluation of the neurological status, only an undifferantiated and coarse estimation is possible. On later performed examinations all scales correlate sufficiently with outcome; this is probably due to the fact that the patients examined in this study were comatose primarily. The outcome was fatal or poor in more than 60% of the cases. Obviously, after many days, many patients assessed with the various scales attained only a low score, which as expected should correlate well with a poor outcome. On the whole the Innsbruck Coma Scale proved to be the best grading for the early evaluation and differentiation of the clinical status as well as for prognostic considerations.

Literature:
1. Hilz,H.J. et al.:Koma-Skalen im Vergleich.In Schwerpunkte neurologischer Intensiv-medizin, Perimed Verlag, 1991; 112-117.
2. Hilz,H.J. et al.::Vergleich von 3 Koma-Skalen und 4 Koma-Scores miteinander und mit der GOS.Intensiv- und Notfallmedizin, 1991;28:398.

70

The Value of Thallium-201-Imaging in Cerebral Lesions: A Comparative Study with Autoradiography and MRI.

Maier-Hauff K, Barzen G, Gottschalk H,
Dept. of Neurosurgery and Radiology, UKRV, FU Berlin,
Augustenburger Platz 1, 1000 Berlin 65, Germany

Indroduction: The outcome of glioma surgery remains unsatisfactory despite of the introduction of MRI and of microsurgical techniques. Therefore the employment of other management processes for the detection of cerebral lesions and therapy control after surgery and radiation therapy were promoted. The results of different investigators (1, 2, 3) were the reason of our examinations having found out:
1. The uptake of 201 Thallium in cerebral tumors reflects viable tumor cells (2).
2. The uptake is more in viable tumor cells than in necrotic cells (2).
3. The uptake is related to cell growth rates (1, 2, 3).

Method: In a study with 48 patients aged 28 - 74 years, 28 men and 20 women, the value of 201-Thallium(TI) ECT was tested. In a second step autoradiographic examinations in microscopic sections were performed comparing the TI 201 uptake in cerebral lesions with the histological result of the processes. 201 TI-ECT was performed 20 min. p.c. (78 MBq) using CT analoge sections. Regions of interest were determined for calculation of the tumor/tissue ratio measuring the TI uptake in normal tissue, tumor or necrotic areas as well as in residual tissue or in tumor recurrence regions.

Results: In low grade gliomas we found a low uptake or no uptake of TI 201 with a quotient of 1 to 2 in contrast to the high grade gliomas showing a high uptake with a quotient of 11. In two patiens residual tumor tissue was detected after surgery only in the TI 201 ECT although CT and MRI showed no pathological signs. The autoradiographic method gives the possibility to see more details making tissue specific differentiations within the tumor e.g. necrosis, cell accumulation, cysts. Comparing the tissue uptake with the autoradiographic findings we saw a good correspondance in both methods except one case of a pituitary adenoma.

Conclusions: 201-TI-ECT is able to detect and differentiate cerebral lesions. Normal brain tissue has no tracer aputake. Tumor cells accumulate 201 TI different. Low grade gliomas have a low tracer uptake in contrast to the malignant gliomas, meningeomas and metastases having a high TI-uptake (rarely low uptake). In contrast to other methods 201 TI shows a therapeutic response concerning residual tumor tissue, tumor recurrence, tumor necrosis and brain swelling. It is desirable in the future to work out with TI 201-ECT a surgical, irradiation and chemotherapeutical concept in the treatment of cerebral gliomas in order to verify the therapeutical response.

References:

1. Elligsen J D, Thompson J E, Frey H E, Kruuv J (1974) Correlation of (Na+-K+)-ATPase activity with growth of normal and transformed cells. Exptl Cell Res 87: 233 -240

2. Kaplan W D, Takvorian T, Morris J H, Rumbaugh C L, Connolly B T, Atkins H L (1987) Thallium-201 brain tumor imaging: A comparative study with pathologic correlation J Nucl Med 28: 47 - 52

3. Kasarov L B, Friedman H (1974) Enhanced Na+-K+-activated adenosine triphosphatase activity in transformed fibroblasts Cacer Res 34: 1862 - 1865

71

123I-IBZM-SPECT IN WILSON'S DISEASE

J. Schwarz[1], K. Tatsch[2], G. Arnold[1], C. Trenwalder[1], J. Scherer[3], C.M. Kirsch[2], WH. Oertel[1]

[1] Dept. of Neurology, Klinikum Grosshadern, Ludwig-Maximilians-University, Munich, Germany and BMFT Research Program Munich "Parkinson's disease and other basal ganglia disorders"
[2] Division of Nuclear Medicine, Dept. of Radiology, Klinikum Grosshadern, Ludwig-Maximilians-University, Munich, Germany
[3] Dept. of Psychiatry, Bezirkskrankenhaus Haar, Munich, Germany

In neuropathological studies of Wilson's disease patients the basal ganglia, especially the striatum, are the primary site of copper deposition in the brain. On the other hand the striatum has the highest density of dopamine D2 receptors in the CNS, at least in rats. Therefore, decreased striatal dopamine D2 recepotor binding may reflect copper related striatal neuronal pathology. ^{123}I-Iodobenzamide-Single Photon Emission Computed Tomography (^{123}I-IBZM-SPECT) is a nuclear medicine technique to investigate srtiatal dopamine D2 receptor binding in vivo. The aim of this study was to investigate whether reduction of ^{123}I-IBZM binding to the basal ganglia would correlate to neurological symptoms in 17 patients with biochemically proven Wilson's disease under long term therapy.

The diagnosis of Wilson's disease was confirmed by characteristic biochemical and ophthalmological findings. 16 patients were treated with D-penicillamine (DPA, 600 to 2000 mg daily) and one patient with zinc (160 mg daily). Five neurological symptoms (dysarthria, ataxia, tremor, rigidity/bradykinesia and chorea/dystonia) were semiquantitatively assessed. The severity of each symptom was scored from 0 (absent) to 3 (severe). The individual scores were than added up resulting in an overall "clinical score".
^{123}I-IBZM-SPECT was performed two hours after i.v. injection of 185 MBq ^{123}I-IBZM. Transverse images were reconstructed by filtered backprojection (Butterworth filter). Specific ^{123}I-IBZM was assessed by a basal ganglia to frontal cortex ratio (BG/FC), which was calculated using the region of interest technique.

The ratio of basal ganglia to frontal cortex was 1.57 ± 0.04 (mean ± SD; n = 5, mean age = 27.8 years, range 25 to 34 years) in five age matched controls. On statistical analysis we observed an almost linear correlation of reduction of ^{123}I-IBZM binding and severity of neurological symptoms under long-term therapy assessed by clinical score at the time of ^{123}I-IBZM-SPECT (correlation coefficient: -0.84, p < 0.01).

Neuropathological findings in Wilson's disease include lesions in the basal ganglia, cerebellum, myelinated fibre bundles, claustrum, red nucleus, subthalamic nucleus, minor cortical changes, and abnormalities of the blood vessels. In most cases the major lesion was within the putamen presenting as increased cellularity mainly due to proliferation of astrocytes. A reduction of ^{123}I-IBZM binding correlates to the severity of neurological symptoms in patients with Wilson's disease under long-term therapy at the time of investigation. This may either reflect a reduction of dopamine D2 receptor densities or an altered state of receptor affinity.

It remains to be prospectively studied, whether ^{123}I-IBZM-SPECT may be used as a predictive or monitoring procedure for the efficacy of the presently available or a new therapy in Wilson's disease of central nervous system or may allow to detect a preclinical striatal lesion in Wilson's disease patients.

72

H-REFLEX OF THE VASTUS MEDIALIS MUSCLE: A NEW DIAGNOSTIC TOOL IN THE TREATMENT OF RUPTURES OF THE ANTERIOR CRUCIATE LIGAMENT:

Wißmeyer, Th; Hülser, P.J.; Kutter, T.; Kinzl, L.

From the Departments of Orthopedic Surgery and Neurology, University Hospital, Ulm, FRG

In assessing the treatment results of the torn anterior cruciate ligament (ACL), up to now the greatest importance has been attached to mechanical stability.
Despite progress in surgical techniques of reconstruction and/or repair of the ruptured ACL clinical results have not always been satisfactory and many questions about this frequently injured ligament are yet to be answered [3].
In order to test not only the passive but also the functional stability of the knee joint, it is necessary to obtain information about the control system of the muscles of the thigh. Therefore, the neurophysiological function of mechanoreceptors in the ACL concerning motion-control and the diagnosis and therapy of ACL-trauma has come increasingly into focus.
Since the early 1980s Johansson and co-workers have investigated the effects of mechanoreceptors in the ACL on the fusimotor-muscle-spindle system (for review see [1]).
To demonstrate impaired function of these receptors, a new and non-invasive method has been developed, wich uses changes in motor-neuron-excitability in quadriceps-muscles during external streching of the ACL. It is well known since the work of Paillard - 1955 that the H-reflex represents an objective criterion to measure the excitability of motoneurons.
In a fixed postion of the leg (35 degrees knee-flexion and 135 degrees hip-flexion) the maximal amplitude of the H-reflex of the vastus medialis muscle is recorded by stimulating the femoral nerve in the groin using changing intensity at the stimulus-frequency of 0.2 Hertz. Adhesive surface electrodes have been used for both stimulation and recording. Custom designed equipment for the experiment assures a relaxed and reproducable position of the lower extremity as well as a constant and well defined pull at the knee joint resulting in anterior forward stress of the proximal tibia.
In 25 patients with suspected rupture of the ACL on one side, the amplitude of the H-reflex was recorded with and without anterior displacement force (F=220N). 20 healthy volunteers were used as a control group.
The amplitude of the H-reflex during stretch of the ACL tended to decrease in patients without injury to the ACL, or in control persons without injury to the ACL. In contrast the amplitude of the H-reflex tended to increase in patients with a ruptured ACL. The proportional changes of the amplitudes between the two groups are statistically significantly different (p less than 0.05).
In our opinion this demonstrates that:
  1) Stimulation of receptors in the ACL leads to inhibition of motoneurons of the quadriceps muscle.
  2) This method allows the evaluation of the neurophysiological function of the intact and ruptured ACL.

References

1. Johansson H, Sjölander P, Soika P (1991) Receptors in the knee joint - ligaments and their role in the biomechanics of the joint. Biomed Engineering 18: 341-368

2. Paillard J (1955) Réflexes et régulations d'origine proprioceptive chez l'homme. Etude neurophysiologique et neuropsychologique. Arnette, Paris

3. Wroble RR, Brand RA (1990) Paradoxes in the history of the anterior cruciate ligament. Clin Orthop 259: 183-191

73

L-DOPA DRUG MONITORING IN PARKINSONIAN PATIENTS

H Baas[1], L Demisch[2], S Harder[3], PA Fischer[1]
[1]Dept. of Neurology, [2]Dept. of Psychiatry
[3]Dept. of Clin.Pharmacology
University of Frankfurt/M, FRG

Complications such as fluctuations, dyskinesias and lack of therapeutic response to L-dopa (NR) are a frequent problem in longterm therapeutic management of Parkinson's disease (PD). Most of them can be summarized under the term of so called L-dopa longterm syndrome (LLS). Influence of peripheral/central pharmacokinetic factors or central pharmacodynamic factors on pathogenesis of those longterm complications is a matter of controversial diskussion.

If peripheral pharmacokinetic factors play an essential role in their pathogenesis, L-dopa drug monotoring might be useful for their management and L-dopa slow release preparations might gain therapeutic value. A serie of studies including an overall of 105 pats. has been performed in our dept. to elucidate pathogenesis of lonterm complications and to determinate the value of L-dopa drug monitoring in PD.

In all pats. single dose studies had been performed under standardized conditions: 100/mg L-dopa/benserazide was given p.o., motor response was measured by CURS and L-dopa plasma concentration (LPC) was measured by HPLC (Baruzzi et al.). All pats. had been fasting and withdrawn from all medication at least 12 hrs. before starting the trial. The examinations had been performed in 15min intervalls over 3 hrs.. Despite marked differences in their motor response we found no differences in pharmacokinetics between de novo, motoric stable, fluctuating (wearing off), and extremely dyskinetic pats. (each group n=10, pats. with severe paroxysmal on/off phenomena excluded). With reference to literature there were no differences to normal volunteers either. In contrast to normal resorption in these pats. in 11 NR-pats. mean L-dopa resorption was significantly delayed (low C_{max}, delayed t_{max}) whereas AUC and plasma elimination parameters were identical to fluctuating and stable pats..

For clarification of the mechanisms leading to delayed resorption in NR-pats., in 2x10 pats. (10 responder, 10 non responder) gastrointestinal emptying was measured by $^{99}Tc^m$-scintigraphy. Pats. were fasting and $^{99}Tc^m$ was applied in a small volume of porridge. Simultaneously LPC after 100/25mg L-dopa/benserazide p.o. were measured in 15min intervalls. Correlation between gastrointestinal emptying time and parameters of L-dopa resorption was found. Delayed L-dopa resorption as well as delayed gastrointestinal emptying could be related to clinical NR.

After peripheral/intestinal acute or chronic DA-receptor blockade by domperidone mean L-dopa resorption could be significantly ($p < 0.05$) accelerated in 14 unselected PD-pats. This improvement occured immediately after first domperidone dose. Nevertheless in a subgroup of 5 NR-pats. where most striking improvement of L-dopa resorption was found, this improvement did not correlate with an adaequate improvement in motor response (measured by CURS). In those pats. additional non dopaminergic neurotransmitter deficits might play a limiting role and prevent major clinical benefit.

Apart from our own studies delayed or aberratic L-dopa resorption was found by Deleu et al. in pats. with severe paroxysmal on/off phenomena.

In conclusion L-dopa drug monitoring might be of some usefulness in pats. with severe paroxysmal on/off phenomena and in so called non responders. But it has to be taken into consideration, that at least in the latter group also other factors such as nondopaminergic neurotransmitter deficits might play an important role.

Reference list on request.

74

REVERSAL OF SPASTICITY AFTER LONG-TERM TREATMENT WITH INTRATHECAL BACLOFEN

J. Dressnandt, A. Konstanzer, B. Conrad
Neurologic Department of the Technical University Munich

The effect of the long-term application of intrathecal baclofen in patients suffering from severe spasticity is not yet known. Within the first year the baclofen dose has to be increased in some patients. This has been reported elsewhere. We have treated 60 patients with spasticity due to multiple sclerosis (MS), spinal or cerebral trauma and drug intoxication (Edrul) with intrathecal baclofen. All patients improved under therapy. When the intrathecal baclofen was reduced then the spasticity and spasms rerturned in most patients but in three, where even after discontinuation of baclofen the spasticity remained improved. At the same time there was a slight increase in paraplegia, irrespective of intrathecal baclofen. Therefore, in some cases there is a change in spinal or supraspinal mechanisms causing spasticity. The reason for this is not clear. One can speculate three mechanisms: 1) The continuous suppression of the calcium influx may change the quantity of the synaptic connections and therefore the plus symptoms of the spasticity are reduced. 2) Baclofen may be toxic to spinal structures. 3) Since we have observed this so far only in MS patients the improvement in spasticity could be due to structural and physiological alterations in central nervous system structures due to MS.

After long term intrathecal application of baclofen it seems useful to try to reduce the baclofen dose, to see if it is still needed.

75

Predictive monitoring in combination therapy of malignant gliomas

Bogdahn U., Jäger A., Richter J.[Θ] Krone A.[≈], Dekant A., Beck A., Pfeufer B. Deptm's. of Neurology , Neurosurgery[≈] and Radiotherapy[Θ], University of Würzburg, Würzburg, F.R.G.

INTRODUCTION. Clinical therapy of patients with high grade gliomas normally consists of surgery, radiotherapy and chemotherapy. Unfortunately, only a minority of patients respond to either radiotherapy and/or chemotherapy, despite an enormous effort to design chemotherapy protocols tailored specificly for brain neoplasms. Numerous approaches have been proposed to predict treatment response of brain tumor patients in vitro, in order to safe prospective non-responders from the unspecific toxicity of a non-efficacious therapy or to offer them experimental alternatives. A shortcoming of all previous predictive methods was their inability to handle drug combinations or the combination of chemotherapy with radiotherapy, schedules practiced in the clinics. We have therefore focussed on designing a new *in vitro* method for evaluation of multi modal treatment interactions, based upon clinical and *in vitro* pharmacokinetics of individual drugs, as well as clinically relevant radiobiological dosimetry.

METHODS: Glioma cell cultures were established from biopsy specimen, passaged and characterized as described before. In vitro chemotherapy was performed with exposure doses calculated from *in vitro* and *in vivo* pharmacokinetic data, for 2 hrs exposure times, experiments were performed with monolayer cultures in 96well-microplate dishes. *In vitro* radiotherapy (0.26 to 4 Gy single dose application) was performed with a standard clinical ^{60}Co radiotherapy unit - a complete *in vitro* dosimetry was performed using thermoluminescence detectors. *In vitro* treatments were performed in sequence (drug A followed by drug B/radiotherpy, and vice versa) . After therapy, tumor cells were allowed to grow for approx. 4 to 5 doubling times, finally a ^{3}H-Thymidin incorporation assay was performed to assess DNA-synthesis as an indirect parameter of cell proliferation.

MATHEMATICAL MODEL: Data points of single treatment arms were approximated by standard probit function, from these a theoretical anticipated additive response surface was created for the interference. Combination experiment data points were then approximated by a generalized probit function to describe an experimental response surface. Finally, local additivity α was derived from the difference between the theoretical additive interaction and the experimentally derived interaction - results are shown as a three dimensional graphic displays, response surfaces may be cut liberally in all three planes (isobole analysis) , significant supra- or sub-additive effects are graphically outlined - correlation coefficients are given for each analysis. (Turbo Pascal 6.0, 80486 Intel processor, graphic display on HPGL-File).

RESULTS AND COMMENTS: The results of different interactions are presented in detail - general results, however, are as follows: (1) this method allows *in vitro* evaluation of multi modal therapy in malignant gliomas with a comparatively low cost/time effort and statistical relevant analysis, (2) the method discriminates "active" and "inert" interactive partners, (3) radio-and chemotherapy may be simulated with equally high standard statistics, (4) this method is the only presented so far, allowing description of local additivity α, which is very important in asymmetrical interactive combinations, (5) although these early results are preliminary, each tumor displays individual patterns for interactive responses, (6) for certain combinations the sequence of treatment is of importance. The clinical validation of this new approach is still pending, as is the finding of a substantially supra-additive combination therapy for malignant gliomas.

76

THE MANAGEMENT OF PRIMARY CEREBRAL LYMPHOMA
Strik H., Müller B., Krauseneck P., Bogdahn U., Richter E.

We reviewed 33 HIV-negative patients with primary cerebral lymphomas treated at the department of neurology of the University of Würzburg since 1978. No systemic manifestation has been observed, four patients had initial or secondary ocular manifestation. Diagnosis was established by resection in 12 patients, by biopsy in 13 cases, 5 times by CSF cytology and 3 times at autopsy only.

While in most series in the literature men predominate slightly, in our group women are nearly twice as common as men. The range of ages varies from 19 to 77 years, most of the patients being 50 to 70 years old. As clinical symptoms focal neurologic signs were seen in 26 cases, neuropsychiatric disorders in 23 cases, 6 patients presented with seizures. The proportion of long term survivors (> 2 years) was approximately constant at 1/3 and did not show an apparent dependency of treatment, age, sex, symptomatology and even not of histology. According to the Kiel classification 10 tumors were classified as low grade, 11 as high grade and 12 remained unclassifiable. All were B-cell lymphomas.

A positive CSF cytology proved to be an important prognostic factor. Half of the 28 examined patients had malignant cells in the CSF initially, a total of 24/28 (86%) at any time of the course of the disease. The prognosis was significantly better for patients without initial CSF manifestation. In some cases relapses could be detected in a very early stage by positive CSF cytology.

No standardised therapy has been applied. Because of unknown diagnosis or acute distress six patients did not receive any specific therapy and died within short time. Due to the infiltrating growth resection can not serve for a better outcome of the patients. All of the long term survivors were not operated. There is no better outcome with combined radio- chemotherapy (RT/CHT) in relation to radiotherapy (RT) alone. However, it has to be taken into account that in the first study years standard therapy was RT alone and chemotherapy (CHT) was only administered in case of relapse. Therefore patients in the RT group are positively selected never having had a relapse. The negative selection for the CHT group is demonstrated by the very short survival times of 4 of the 5 patients treated after relapse only. However, also in one of these patients several relapses could successfully be treated by Ara-C and she is alive now for more than 5 years in complete remission. Using CHT in an adjuvant setting, the 6 patients treated in the last years clearly lived longer, 4 being still alive.

The median survival time in the whole group is 16 months. In the 26 patients with any completed treatment the median survival is 26 months. We never used high-dose chemotherapy schedules in first line.

In the international literature one outstanding result is reported by de Angelis et al. from Memorial Sloan Kettering Cancer Centre: In a prospective study with 32 patients they achieved a median survival time of 48 months with a standardised treatment consisting of whole brain RT, intrathecal methotrexate (MTX), corticosteroids and pre- radiation systemic high-dose MTX plus two series high-dose Ara-C after irradiation. They did not report on neurotoxic side effects, although (severe) leucoencephalopathy is a well known complication of high-dose MTX-doses, at least if administered simultaneously or after RT, what was avoided by these authors. In our hands Ara-C was as effective as MTX for intrathecal treatment and was well tolerated also after RT.

Conclusion:

PCL should be suspected in multiple or deep-seated midline lesions with homogeneous contrast enhancement and diffuse margin. A CSF cytology should be done as early as possible, because the frequency of malignant cells is high. Routine slit lamp examination is advisable since approx. 20% show infiltration of the vitrous.

Diagnosis should be established as rapidly as possible, usually by stereotaxic biopsy, and any delay by extensive search for a possible primary must be avoided.

Standard treatment consists in whole brain irradiation (28-30 x 1,8 Gy) plus intrathecal chemotherapy with MTX or Ara-C.

According to the literature and to our own experience adjuvant CHT is effective and improves the survival data. However, the ideal chemotherapy combination is yet to be found.

77

Follow-up study of patients who suffered from bacterial meningoencephalitis

B. Zahner, H. Stefan, H. Feistel, M.J. Hilz, M. Harrer, B.Neundörfer

Neurology department of the University of Erlangen-Nuremberg (Director Prof. Dr. med. B. Neundörfer)

104 patients with bacterial meningitis (n=34) or bacterial meningoencephalitis (n=70) were examined. The initial diagnosis was set up by regarding clinical symptoms, inflammatory changes in lumbar puncture, electroencephalography (EEG) and imaging devices. 46 patients answered questionnaires at least 6 months after acute onset of the disease, 30 patients were examined as outpatients. A neurological examination, a neuropsychological examination (standardized Reischies test), EEG and 99-m-Tc-Hm-PAO SPECT-examination of the brain were performed. Moreover the patients were requested to give details of possible further symptoms.
Median age was 49 years for the patients who suffered from meningoencephalitis and 27 years for the patients who suffered from meningitis.
Meningoencephalitis was caused most frequently by Streptococcus pneumonia, other germs were less frequent. In 40% of the patients detection of the germ that caused the infection was not possible. In 22 (31.5%) of all patients who suffered from bacterial meningoencephalitis a purulent process in the area of the head (e.g. chronical otitis media) was the underlying disease, 3 patients (4.3%) suffered from a purulent spondylodiscitis that caused encephalitis. Letality was 22.8% in bacterial meningoencephalitis and 6.6% in meningitis.
The questionnaires showed that about 30% of the questioned persons with encephalitis and 26% of the persons who had meningits did not have any further complaints. The rest of these patients still suffers from different subjective complaints such as headache (about 32% after encephalitis and 37%! after meningitis), dizziness (38% after encephalitis and 44% after meningitis) or global memory deficits (48% after encephalitis and 22% after meningitis). 30% (9 patients) of the examined patients did not show significant abnormalities in all examinations, 46.6% (14 patients) had pathological SPECT-examinations and pathological findings in at least one of the other examinations. In 3 patients (10%) the examinations were not significantly abnormal except for a pathological SPECT. In 6 (20%) patients we found a Theta or Theta/Delta Focus in EEG localized at the same area as a hypoperfusion in SPECT. On the whole, more than 50% of the patients had abnormalities of perfusion in SPECT. It has to be taken into consideration that not all perfusion deficits must be due to the cerebral infection, but at least some of the patients who did not have other vascular diseases or brain abscesses also get perfusion deficits after a severe infection.
10 patients (33%) showed minor neurological deficits (such as symptoms of cranial nerves or not too extensive weakness of limbs on one side), 2 patients (6,7%) had severe deficits such as tetraparesis, global aphasia or organic brain syndrome, the other patients who were examined did not have any neurological deficits. On the whole, only about half of the examined patients did not show abnormalities in the neurological and the neuropsychological examination.
The correlation of technical diagnostic examinations such as SPECT, EEG, CT (performed in some cases) is discussed with the results of the neurological and neuropsychological findings.
Bacterial meningoencephalitis still is a very severe disease, mortality is still high, and, as this study shows, the outcome sometimes shows severe neurologic sequelae. An early appropriate therapy with antimicrobial agents is of great importance.

78

Investigation of hemodynamics in therapy of acute stroke patients

Treib J, Stoll M, Haaß A, Scherer J, Jost V
Departement of Neurology, University of Saarland, W-6650 Homburg/Saar, FRG

During therapy of 52 patients suffering from acute (<12 hours) and non acute cerebral vascular desease (CVD) we performed a 24 resp. 36 hour long-term measurement of cardiac output (CO), heart rate, stroke volume and ejection fraction using a thoracic bioimpedance monitor. Additionally a continuous blood pressure registration was done.
The initial CO of the acute CVD patients was 39% lower compared with the non acute patients. They also showed less variation and no over night decrease of the measured CO values, which we interpret as a sign of an intravascular volume deficit and of diminished cardial capacity.
We performed a hypervolemic hemodilution in the acute patients (n=6) by volume application. First we infused in 45 minutes a loading dose of 500 ml 10% hydroxyethylstarch 200/0.5 and 500 ml electrolyte solution followed by infusion of the double amount in 24 hours.
14 of the 39 patients with non acute CVD were treated in the same way. Patients showing signs of manifest heart failure were excluded. More than half of these patients showed a fast 20%-increase of CO, which persisted for about 3 hours, followed by a slowly decrease. This enhancement of CO was mostly caused by an increased stroke volume, essential changes of blood pressure couldn't be found.
The acute patients without signs of heart failure reacted in the same way. In acute patients showing discrete or moderate heart failure (NYHA II-III) no increase of cardiac output could be found. This cannot be interpreted as a beginning cardial decompensation, but as a missing ability to improve heart performance, because we didn't see a hemodynamic deterioration in any patient. Only an additional fast digitalisation resp. application of catecholamines in selected cases slowly improved the hemodynamic situation. An isovolemic hemodilution performed in 25 patients failed in improving hemodynamic paremeters.
In 7 healthy patients we examined the circadian rhythm by 24 hour long-term measurement of the hemodynamic parameters described above. We found a clearly over night decrease of CO and blood pressure, which we interpret partly as signs of hypovolemia. Together with an simultaneous increase of hematocrit this may be a reason for the high rate of ischemic cerebral infarctions in the early morning hours.
Our results stress the importance of an quick compensation of hypovolemia in patients suffering from acute cerebral infarction, in order to improve perfusion of the ischemic penumbra by increasing cardial preload and so CO.

79

Strategies in Endovascular Treatment of Spontaneous Cavernous Sinus Fistulas

H.C.Nahser(1), D.Kühne(1), E. Berg-Dammer(2), H. Henkes(1), E. Möbius(2)

(1) Abteilung für Neuroradiologie, (2)Klinik für Neurologie
Alfried-Krupp-Krankenhaus Essen
Alfried Krupp Straße 21 D-4300 Essen

Symptomatic spontaneous cavernous sinus fistulas in 56 patients have been referred to our institution.Spontaneous cavernous sinus fistulas are classified according to Barrow. Type A fistulas belong to the direct group, whose etiology is that of ruptured cavernous aneurysms. In the remaining 46 dural fistulas of the cavernous sinus wall, which have different arterial supply hormonal influencies are discussed, because onset of symptoms is most common in postmenopausal or pregnant women. Type D with combined external and internal carotid blood supply is dominating. Cortical drainage (7 of 47 in our series), with the possibility of intracranial hemorrhage in the course is in our opinion more often identified with better angiographic equipment. We treated 56 cases, out of which 10 were direct (Type A of the Barrow classification) and 46 were dural arteriovenous fistulas (Type B =9, C =13 and D =24).Concerning the direct fistulas the same treatment approach as in traumatic fistulas was applied. Balloon embolization resulted in 10 selective occlusion of the fistula with clinical and radioanatomical cure. In dural A-V fistulas digital compression of the carotid artery and iugular vein as introduced by Halbach alone provided a control of symptoms in 6 cases. If there was no improvement or ocular disturbances increased and visual loss occurred transarterial embolization of feeding meningeal branches lead to a control of symptoms in 13 and a cure in 17 patients. When there was drainage of the fistula to cortical veins with the high risk of hemorrhage or high ocular pressure was not relieved by particle embolization, a definite closure of the fistula had to be achieved by transvenous coil occlusion (9 cases). Direct catheterization of internal feeders is restricted to cases in which a transvenous approach is not possible.

Barrow DL, Spector RH, Braun IF, Landman JA, Tindall SC, Tindall GT:Classification and treatment of carotid-cavernous sinus fistulas.JNeurosurg 1985;62:248-256.

Halbach VV, Higashida RT, Hieshima GB, Reicher M, Norman D, Newton TH.Dural fistulas involving the cavernous sinus: results of treatment in 30 patients.Radiology 1987;163:437-442.

80

VISUAL FIELD INDICES FOR LESIONS OF THE CENTRAL VISUAL PATHWAYS

F. Dannheim*, St. Wessel**

*Dept. of Ophtalmology, University of Hamburg

**Dept. of Neurology, Heidberg General Hospital, Hamburg

The database PERIDATA provides a number of new indices by calculating the conformity of values of sensivity in confirmed areas of the central visual field. We applied two of these, one for hemiopic and another one for quadranopic defects, to the OCTOPUS G1 normative population (n=836), and to visual fields in lesions of the chiasm (n=106), the optic tract (n=34), of supra-geniculate lesions (n=36), and fields in optic neuritis (n=75).

The hemi-index was abnormal in 50, the quadrant-index in 53 healthy eyes (specifity 94%). 144 of 150 fields with hemiopic defects due to lesions of the chiasm or further central pathways presented with a pathological hemi-index (sensivity 96%). All 6 missed fields had only mild hemiopic alterations and a pathological quadrant-index. From 55 abnormal fields in optic neuritis, only 4 showed a moderately elevated hemi-index, whereas 12 had an abnormal quadrant-index due to nasal nerve fibre defects. The separation of the different clinical entities with these indices is demonstrated by ROC curves. The two indices obviously facilitate the interpretation of visual fields and are qualified to control the therapy of lesions of central visual pathwayes.

Therapy monitoring

81

Tardive dystonia in a study population of 450 patients presenting with focal or segmental dystonia

I. Kühne, A.O. Ceballos-Baumann, B. Conrad

Neurologische Klinik, Technische Universität München

The concept of tardive dyskinesia involves three or more distinct syndromes: 1. classical tardive (orobuccolingual) dyskinesia, 2. **tardive dystonia** and 3. tardive akathisia. By definition tardive dyskinesia syndromes occur during or after exposure (6 months is currently advocated as cut-off time) to neuroleptic type drugs (more specific: dopamine receptor blockers). Since tardive dystonia may phenomenologically mimic idiopathic dystonia diagnosis depends on the history about the onset of dystonia in relation to exposure to dopamine receptor blockers.

Data on the characteristics, course as well as causative agents are scarce on larger patient collectives with tardive dystonia.

We reviewed the clinical data of 450 patients referred for the evaluation and treatment of focal/segmental dystonia. The data were prospectively collected with a standardized questionaire. 73 patients were categorized at the time of the initial presentation as having had definite or likely exposure to dopamine receptor blockers in the previous 6 months or during the onset of the dystonia. The drug history was then analysed in this group of 73 patients contacting general practitioners, tracing records and reexamining patients.

In a great proportion of this "likely tardive group" the relationship between onset of dystonia and exposure to dopamine receptor blockers remained unclear (44 of 73 patients). A definite history of exposure to dopamine receptor blockers could be documented in 29 of the 73 patients (age at onset: mean 41,4; 23-73; 15 female, 14 male). 14 patients had been treated for psychosis with dopamine receptor blockers. Only in 3 of this 14 patients onset of the tardive dystonia prompted a change to clozapine. Patients displayed following focal/segmental dystonias: 3 anterocollis, 3 axial dystonia, 6 blepharospasm, 4 spasmodic dysphonia, 9 oromandibular dystonia (8 jaw closing type, 1 jaw opening type), 12 retro-torticollis, 1 foot dystonia. 11 patients also had akathisia. No hand dystonia could be ascertained as tardive. Haloperidol (8 patients), fusperilen (7) and fluanxol i.m. (5) could be related most frequently to the onset of the tardive dystonia, but also metoclopropamide (3) and flunarizine (2). A remission of tardive dystonia was observed in one patient 5 months after discontinuing the neuroleptic. Treatment with botulinum toxin of tardive dystonia was less helpful compared to similar patients with idiopathic dystonia.

Exposure to neuroleptic-type drugs as a cause of focal/segmental dystonia is common. Our data indicate that there is little awareness about tardive dystonia as a incapacitating and commonly persisting side effect of the use of dopamine receptor blockers. A more stringent indication for the use of dopamine receptor blockers and a more rapid change to clozapine in those patients who need neuroleptics and who are developing tardive dystonia seems warranted.

82

Computer-Aided Analysis Of Cranial CCT And MRT Images

F.Kruggel and H. Gräfin von Einsiedel
Neurologische Klinik, Klinikum Rechts der Isar
Möhlstrasse 28, 8000 München 80

With the event of new powerful computer equipment recording patient data from different sources onto opto-electronical media and their correlative evaluation became possible.

Our Medical Documentation System (MDS) addresses this problem. It's purpose is to document texts, numerical data, pictures (i.e. X-ray pictures, photos, anatomical and histological preparations), curves (i.e. ECG, EEG, EP) and speech. This software package runs in a network of UNIX-workstations from different vendors using X-Windows R11.5/Motif as an graphical user interface.

Patient data is displayed in a spreadsheet-like manner consisting of patient cases as columns and observed data (i.e. laboratory data, CCT, EMG) as rows. Powerful and generally usable editors for texts, curves and pictures were developed. An underlying spreadsheet and presentation package serves for evaluating data.

Our current work centers on the exploration of specific usages for the general tools. In neurology there is a special interest in correlating brain lesions with clinical observations. The exact topographical analysis of brain stem or basal ganglia lesions is hard to fulfil by visual means. On the basis of well-known anatomical maps a series of screen masks were developed which can interactively be adapted to actual CT slices. These maps contain informations of anatomical locations and vascular territories.

In a retrospective study a series of MRT scans of patients with stereotactically produced brain lesions were analysed for their exact anatomical location. MRT and CCT images where input either on-line (over network), off-line (by tape) or by redigitising films using a high-resolution video camera. Lesions were described numerically by location, extent and completeness.

This way a fast, standardised and anatomical exact analysis of CT slices is possible. The underlying database is user-definable, so additions and modifications can be made at any time. A transposition to similar localisation problems in other regions seems possible.

83

Interrater agreement for CT scans of patients with lacunar infarcts and leuko-araiosis

R. Schneider, R. Kluge, K. Willmes
Department of Neurology, Klinikum RWTH,
D-5100 Aachen, Germany

Introduction: For the CT diagnosis of lacunar infarcts, various research groups have developed various criteria which still are a matter of controversy. Morphological criteria for CT scans have also been described for the diagnosis of leuko-araiosis. According to our experience assessments of lacunar infarcts and leuko-araiosis by different observers exhibit considerable differences with respect to specific rating criteria. This prompted study on the agreement between raters who are to assess lesions of the white matter.

Methods and Results: Seventy-four CT scans from patients with lacunar syndromes were presented to 10 raters, most of them experienced in neuroradiology. The attributes to be judged were: lacunar infarcts (yes/no), leuko-araiosis (decreased density of the cerebral white matter) (yes/no), cortical atrophy (yes/no), and normal (yes/no). The raters were given no information on the subjects history or clinical findings. However, a rigid definition of lacunar infarcts was administered (see Discussion). The chance corrected kappa-coefficients were 0.651 for decreased density, 0.445 for lacunar infarcts and 0.206 for cortical atrophy. Taking into consideration the attribute cortical atrophy, the kappa-coefficient for the attribute normal was 0.330, and without taking cortical atrophy into consideration, it was 0.523.

Discussion: Our results underscore that there still exist substantial rating differences even in the presence of rigid definitions and their application in only one department. Our conclusion is: in the absence of a uniform definition of lacunar infarcts any study on this subject will be speculative. Studies of lacunar infarcts and of leuko-araiosis should be based on clear definitions in order to garanty a minimum level of interrater agreement. For practical reasons we suggest that CT scan evaluation should be based on the consensus judgement of at least three experienced raters. Statistical analysis of all parameters measured should only be based on the data of those patients whose CT scans were evaluated consistently by these experienced raters. Furthermore, we suggest the following criteria for the diagnosis of lacunar infarcts: maximum diameter less than 10 mm, round or ovally shaped, located in the basal ganglia, the lower corona radiata, the capsula interna, and the brainstem. Patients which have atrophic changes in CT should not be included in studies about lacunae or leuko-araiosis.

Schneider R, Kluge R, Willmes K (1991) Interrater agreement for CT scans of patients with lacunar infarcts and leuko-araiosis. Acta Neurol Scand 84: 527-530

84

Prognostic value of MEP and SSEP in patients with chronic UMN lesions after stroke
KM Stephan, J Netz and V Hömberg

Neurological Therapy Center, Heinrich Heine University,
Düsseldorf, Germany

The purpose of this study was to investigate the prognostic value of Motor Evoked Potentials (MEP) and Sensory Evoked Potentials (SSEP) in comparison to that of a detailed clinical examination in patients with chronic upper motor neurone lesions after stroke.

55 patients after stroke were investigated. Mean age was 50 years (16 to 80 years) and mean duration of disease 15 months (1 to 163 months). Motor function, tone, surface sensory modalities and joint position sense were tested seperately for the affected hand, arm and leg. For assessment of motor function a detailed motor score was used (1). Motor evoked potentials were obtained from thenar and abductor hallucis muscles bilaterally using magnetoelectrical stimulation. Cortical somatosensory evoked potentials were recorded after median and tibial nerve stimulation.

All patients were admitted to a community based neurological therapy center. Clinical examination was repeated at the end of therapy. Mean time between first and final examination was 5 months (including time before admission).

Motorscores were the best predictors for motor function after therapy for hand, arm and leg function. Joint position sense had an additonal prognostic value for fine motor function of the hand. MEP and SSEP had a positive correlation with motor outcome, correlation values for both techniques were higher for upper than for lower extremities. In general MEP showed closer correlations with final motor scores than SSEP, which is in line with observations in patients with acute stroke (2). Regression analysis however revealed an additional prognostic value of MEP only for hand function.

12 patients had only slightly impaired hand function before therapy: all six with normal MEP and SSEP showed further improvement, four of them a 'full recovery'. Only three of the six patients with similar clinical data but pathological MEP and/or SSEP improved further, none showing 'full recovery' As MEP are thought to investigate the intactness of direct corticospinal projections, it is likely, that their intact state is a necessary but not sufficient element for full recovery of fine finger movements.

In conclusion in patients with chronic upper motor neurone syndrome after stroke MEP and SSEP can help to explore the (pathophysiological) scope for further improvement of fine finger function but not predict its exact scale.

References:
1. Hömberg V, Stephan KM, Netz J (1991) Transcranial stimulation of motor cortex in upper motor neurone syndrome: its relation to the motor deficit. Electroenceph Clin Neurophysiol 81: 377 - 388
2. Macdonnel RAL, Donnan A, Bladin PF (1989) A comparison of somatosensory evoked and motor evoked potentials in stroke. Ann Neurol 25: 68 - 73

85

HABITUATION OF THE BLINK REFLEX - PROGNOSTIC SIGN FOR PATIENTS IN THE VEGETATIVE STATE (APALLIC SYNDROME)

P.W. Schönle, D. Schwall

Forschungsinstitut für Rehabilitationsneurologie und Neuropsychologie, Kliniken Schmieder, D-7753 Allensbach

Early assessment of prognostic factors in patients with persistent/transient vegetative state appears to be an extraordinary challenge for intensive care neurology and early neurological rehabilitation. While vegetative and sensorimotor functions are important faculties of the central nervous system - quoad vitam - recovery of mental functions are of fundamental significance for the restitution of a truly human, spiritual life and personality.

In order to evaluate returning basic functions of the higher integrative CNS activity in patients with persistent/transient vegetative state or in its remittant stages, a habituation learning paradigm has been applied. Habituation of visually, acoustically, tactually and electrically elicited blink reflexes have been analysed in 8 patients between 14 and 39 years in vegetative state after severe brain damage.

Clinical rating was established by the use of the *Glasgow Coma Scale* (**GCS**), the *Disability Rating Scale* by RAPPAPORT (**DRS**) and the *Koma Remission Scale* (**KRS**) (German working group on early rehabilitation).

Sequences of 10 stimulations were applied in the "awake" patient in three modalities: a) visual (rapid hand movement towards the eyes); b) auditory (hand-clapping); c) tactile (glabella-tapping with reflex hammer).

In addition to the clinical testing procedure electromyographic recordings of the orbicularis oculi muscle were performed under a) visual, b) auditory (bursts of 124 dB SPL/1 kHz), c) tactile (tapping with a triggering hammer), and d) electrical (conventional orbicularis-oculi-reflex) stimulating conditions in order to detect subclinical reactions of the patients and to control the clinical evaluation.

Results of routinely performed visual and auditory evoked potentials (VEP and AEP) were taken into account, when patients showed unresponsiveness to stimulation of one or the other sensory channel.

Preliminary results show significant better habituation in patients with higher levels of consciousness (> 10 pts./GCS; < 20/DCS; > 14/KRS) and improving habituation during the clinical course if improvement of the clinical status resulted. The clinical observations were confirmed by the electrophysiological findings. Fast physiological habituation (FOX 1978, BROWN et al. 1991) found in neurologically intact or recovering subjects contrasted to the persistent eye-lid movements in patients with persistent vegetative state. Patients with occuring habituation demonstrated a better prognosis in terms of restitution of higher cortical functions.

Eye blink habituation tested in various modalities may, therefore, be taken as an early indicator of the restitution of learning capabilities of the CNS. Thanks to the simple applicability and ease of quantification the procedure could turn out to become a valuable clinical screening tool for prognostic assessment of patients in the early stages of vegetative states (apallic syndroms).

References

FOX-JE (1978) Excitatory and inhibitory components of the eyeblink responses to startle evoking stimuli. Electroencephalogr. Clin. Neurophysiol 44(4):490-501

BROWN-P,ROTHWELL-JC,THOMPSON-PD, BRITTON-TC, DAY-DL, MARSDEN-CD (1991) New observations on the normal auditory startle reflex in man. Brain 114:1891-1902

86

Results of a computer aided movement analysis for the therapy control and staging of patients with movement disorders

C. Bischoff, J. Machetanz, B.-U. Meyer, F. Pallmann, B. Conrad

Neurologische Klinik der Technischen Universität München Möhlstr. 28; 8000 München 80; Germany

In patients with movement disorders the common method for staging de novo patients and for monitoring success of therapy is to use rating scales or - in clinical practice - to conduct specific clinical tests, record the essential findings and keep details in mind. As an alternative instrument, we developed and tested a microcomputer (MS-DOS) based system which was designed for the analysis of manual movement disabilities in patients with various motor disorders. The system includes ballistic, pursuit tracking, complex sequential and finger tapping tasks. The standardized test procedure lasted about 40 minutes per subject. The main parameters analyzed were reaction time, movement time, general deviation of the tracker from the target, lag, correlation, tapping rate and a parameter reflecting hypokinetic versus hyperkinetic movement characteristics. The following examples demonstrate possible applications of the computerized movement analysis system:

1. We assessed 30 patients with Parkinson's disease with both, the computer system and the UPD rating scale. The UPD scale includes the Schwab and England scale of activities of daily living. The Schwab and England score was found to correlate better with various parameters measured by the computer system than with any of the subtests of the UPDRS. For example, the computer parameter assessing correlation between tracker symbol and target symbol in pursuit tracking had a coefficient of R=0.67 and the regression was at p<.00005 highly significant. This shows that the computer system catches features of the disease which are clinically relevant and that it may be a useful method for a standardized estimation of manual disability. Because the system does not depend on subjective ratings it can be particularly useful in multicenter studies in order to establish common standards for the staging of manual movement disabilities.

2. It is a major problem in the clinical observation of the long term course of motor disorders that smaller changes in motor disability are extremely difficult to judge. We performed repeated tests in 6 patients with chronic degenerative diseases (HD, PD, LOCA, Friedreich's ataxia) holding the interval between the repetitions to at least 6 months. In all cases deteriorations in the measured parameters were found, although a clear deterioration was noted in the clinical examination in only two patients. In one case (HD) the relatives had even believed in an improvement during the questionable period. The measured extent of motor deterioration was in accordance with the rate of disease progression as could be expected from common clinical knowledge about the different diseases.

3. In individual patients who are not able to give a reliable account of changes in their condition which are related to therapeutical measures, it is important to have an objective criterion for planning therapy. This is particularly relevant in depressed patients who tend to see only negative results of any measures. We assessed a parkinson patient who complained of deterioration of his left hand tremor after a change in medication. The objective measurements disclosed that in fact a right hand improvement of tremor had occurred while the left hand tremor had remained unchanged. Thus, it was possible to identify the patient's complaints as a result of the misinterpreted observation that the tremor expression had become more similar in the two hands.

COMPUTER-ASSISTED VIDEOANALYSIS IN THERAPY CONTROL OF MOVEMENT DISORDERS

Ohlmann D.[1], Krick C.[2], Jäger H.[1], Nachtigall W.[2], Schimrigk K.[1]

[1]Department of Neurology, 6650 Homburg/ Saar
[2]Department of Zoology, 6600 Saarbrücken,
   University of Saarland

Movements and especially movement disorders in neurological patients used to be subjectively described without any quantification. The classification into "spontaneously motor processes (chorea, athetosis, dystonia, i. a.)" and "active movement disorders (ataxia, intension tremor, action myoclonus, i. a.)" already points out the problem: the intermitting occurence, the dependence on activity and the complexity of mimical movements in particular complicate reproducible quantification. So the long-term follow up and the therapy control are difficult.

We developed a method for describing and quantifying movement disorders, consisting of a video camera, a S-VHS-video recorder, a video processor card, a personal computer and special software.

In a standardized trial patients are videotaped after marking the parts affected with white spots (5*5 mm). Sequences must be digitalized in single images with the help of a computer generated time code. The minimal period between is 40 ms and can be variably alterated upwards. 15 images are evaluated "en bloc". The computer localizes the spots (area of interest) and 4 patients with torticollis spasmodicus before and after treatment, 4 patients with tremor (2 parkinson- 1 essential- and one with unknown etiology) and 5 with cerebral ataxia were investigated using the method described above. It was possible to figure the improvement of the dystonic disorders after therapy. The tremor analysis includes the ascertainment of frequency and amplitude. Point-to-point- (finger-to-nose-, a modified findertip-to-fingertip- and knee-to-heel-) manoeuvres were employed in the quantification of the ataxic disorders.

The new developed method allows the graphical evaluation of movements and related disorders. The influence of affective amplification and circardiane rhythm still remains a problem. Nevertheless an optimal long-term follow up and therapy control become possible without stressing the patient. Only a minimal technical and financial expenditure is necessary.

Development of a microcomputer system for therapy control of patients with movement disorders

J. Machetanz, J. Forster, C. Bischoff, B.U. Meyer, B. Conrad
Neurologische Klinik der Technischen Universität München; Möhlstr. 28; 8000 München 80

Considerable research during recent decades was directed towards an identification and quantification of the characteristic movement disturbances in different movement disorders. However, the results had almost no concrete influence on clinical practice. Several measuring systems that were developed in different laboratories did not find a broad application because the required hardware and the additional personal staff were too expensive for most hospitals. With the appearance of cheap microcomputers and comfortable software tools there is now a base available for low-cost and easy to use systems. Therefore, we have developed software needing no hardware except a 386 MS-DOS computer with a hard disk, 640 KB RAM and a Microsoft-compatible mouse. Because all movement data are acquired using the mouse no IO- or AD-boards are necessary. The program is written in Borland Turbo Pascal Ver. 6 and includes the Turbo Vision user surface which uses pull-down menus and which includes a hypertext help facility. The program is structured into five main modules: A password protected patient databank holding personal and clinical data, the acquisition module, the analysis module, the result presentation module and the setup module.

There are four different paradigms that can be assessed with the program: pursuit tracking, ballistic tasks, complex sequential tasks and finger tapping. Within these paradigms various variables (for example movement pattern, velocity, amplitude, frequency etc. in pursuit tracking) can be manipulated. Data acquisition can be conducted alternatively in two different modes: in the first mode the medical assistant conducting the test defines the paradigm with all variables before each recording. In the second mode a complete test set consisting of various paradigms with any combination of variables can be predefined and saved to a file. When the patient is actually tested, the assistant has only to retrieve this file and can run the complete test without giving any special attention to the paradigms and variables that are used. For data analysis again two different methods are available. First, a waveform editor allows for an inspection of the raw data using different display types and transformations including first and second derivations. The second method is advantageous in clinical environments. It automatically extracts all essential parameters from a complete test set. Important examples of such parameters in pursuit tracking the mean absolute deviation of the tracker waveform from the target, the correlation and lag in the ballistic task reaction time and movement time, in the complex sequential task movement time and in the finger tapping tapping rate. In all tasks except tapping a kinesia parameter was additionally calculated that quantifies hyperkinetic or hypokinetic characteristics of the movements.

Results are displayed using built in diagrams which can also be customized to individual wishes. For example, parameter units can be chosen to be SI units or the parameters can be standardized using normative data. The normative data can be either a large sample of norm subjects of similar age or they can be automatically calculated using a built in algorithm of the age function. Within this algorithm the variables of each standard task are based on a norm group of 78 subjects that were assessed with the standard test set. If the user wants to conduct specific analyses that exceed the capabilities of the built in diagrams he can export the analyzed parameters as well as the original raw data in ASCII files to standard statistics packages or other software.

89

A New Versatile RF Data-Acquisition Module For Tissue Characterisation

•B.Bresser, •W.Thomas, •R.M.Schmitt, *U.Mielke, •H.J.Welsch, +E. Lagler

• Fraunhofer Institute for Bio Medical Engeneering, St. Ingbert, Germany
* Neurology, Medical Shool, University of Saarland, Germany
+ Kretztechnik GmbH, Zipf, Austria

Abstract

The possibility of extracting histological information, especially by backscattered ultrasound is of great interest for the improvement of differential diagnosis using ultrasonic device. In order to evaluate sceletal muscle disease and muscular malfunction a new electronic module for tissue characterisation has been developed and constructed, which is presently under clinical testing. The module integrates a Region-Of-Interest-(ROI-) controller, a transient recorder and an interface to a PC-compatible.

To have no loss of signal-information the system is specially taylored for the **real-time-acquirement**, the storage and the processing of **RF-Data** taken from user-selected ROIs. A 60 MSample digitizing unit is employd to reduce digitization-noise and spectral aliasing. A signal-to-noise ratio of up to 60 dB is reached by a AD conversion depth of 10 Bit. An intermediate memory of 16 MByte integrated in the transient-recorder allows the storage of image-sequences. The number of subsequent frames depends on the frame size. The latter is determined by use of the ROI. The transient-recorder is equipped with an operating system which is controlled by a PC-compatible where the data are transferred to for further processing. The ROI-controller provides a visual control of ROI and is extendible to the definability of several ROIs within one frame. It has been universally designed in order to guarantee a high adaptability to all kinds of US-Scanners used in clinical every-day-life.

The data can be processed and evaluated by a highly sophisticated software especially developed for clinical needs. It includes powerful methods of parametric tissue-classification as well as a high-performance image-data-processing. The parameters obtainable are frequency dependent attenuation, integrated backscatter and the autocorrelation-based determination of scatterer-sizes; the possibilities of general data-processing comprise filtering and 2-D-spectral estimation algorithms. To provide a universal usability of data and results, only well-known data-formats like TIFF or ASCII are used. Results of experiments with phantoms and real muscle-examinations will be presented.

90

Muscle-twitch studies in hypothyroidism

Dillmann, U.; Krämer, G.; Lüder G. and H. C. Hopf

Department of Neurology, University of Mainz, Mainz, FRG

In hypothyroidism contraction and relaxation of isometric muscle twitches are prolonged even if clinical or myographic signs of myopathy are missing. We studied the changes of contractility in hypothyroidsm and their recovery during treatment.

Isometric contractions of the adductor pollicis muscle evoked by ulnar nerve stimulation were studied in 7 hypothyroid patients and a control group of 30 healthy volunteers. Single and double stimuli with intervals of 0.6 to 180 ms were used. Twitch-potentiation was examined by applying 2 Hz stimulati for 50 sec. Recovery of potentiation was tested by single stimuli 10, 30, 60, 120, 180, 240 and 300 sec. afterwards.

The significantly prolonged contraction and relaxation of twitches in hypothyroidism had only little changed one month after administration of thyroid hormones. Six months later, however, there was marked improvement, only the mechanical latency and the contraction time were still slightly prolonged. Thyroid hormone- and thyroid stimulating hormone levels, at that time, were within the normal range.

During repetitive stimulation, the hypothyroid muscle shows a pronounced initial decrease of force, a reduced twitch potentiation which does not reach the initial level during the stimulation phase and a strong potentiation over 5 minutes in the poststimulation period. In the healthy control group, there is a potentiation to + 15% normalizing within 4 minutes. One month later, potentiation of twitch force returned to normal, but the enhanced poststimulation-twitch potentiation was still present. After six month, potentiation normalized within the same time as the control group.

Twitch potentiation during and after low frequency repetitive stimulation is a sensitive test of muscle function during hypothyroid therapy indicating two different pathophysiological processes.

91

A New Treatment Concept for Acute Guillain-Barré Syndrome: Basis for a Multicenter Study

W.F.Haupt*, H.Borberg**, F.Rosenow*

Departments of Neurology (*) and Hemapheresis (**)

University of Cologne, Germany

The Guillain-Barré Syndrome (GBS) is an inflammatory disease of the peripheral nerve leading to discontinuous demyelination of the axon. Its cause is as yet unknown although a large amount of clinical and experimental data suggest an immunological pathogenesis. Since the prognosis of the disease is generally favorable, aggressive treatment is to be advocated.

Numerous treatment trials with steroids have been undertaken with variable dosages but no conclusive positive results have been reported. Plasma exchange treatment has been shown by two large multicenter trials to be effective. Also, a Dutch multicenter trial has shown intravenous immunoglobulins to be more effective than plasma exchange treatment. Therefore, it seems questionable whether further multicenter studies in GBS using conventional plasma exchange will provide any new information.

In our own anecdotal experience, we found that selective adsorption treatment of GBS using a tryptophan adsorption column (TR 350) may be considered an alternative to plasma exchange treatment. Controlled studies with selective adsorption in GBS have not been conducted yet. We treated 27 patients with acute GBS by either conventional plasma exchange (11 patients), selective adsorption against a TR 350 column (7 patients), and a combination of selective adsorption with subsequent IgG treatment (9 patients). We tested the null hypothesis that all three treatment groups showed no significant differences in clinical course, analyzing the following criteria: Impairment at hospital admission, maximal impairment, change of impairment during treatment, and duration to first documented clinical improvement. These variables showed no statistical group differences (P>0.12).

To assess the incidence of complications, we compared the clinical data of 10 patients with conservative treatment alone to 10 patients treated by plasma exchange and to another 10 patients treated by selective adsorption. The three groups were matched for age and degree of maximal disability. The group comparison showed no difference with respect to procedural complications. We gained the impression that plasma exchange and selective adsorption with or without IgG treatment shows similar results.

Our hypotheses are:
1. Selective adsorption may be a treatment alternative to plasma exchange with similar efficacy and with the advantage that the procedure is less stressing for the patient, as the amount of plasma processed is smaller, which has less effect on plasma proteins and the coagulation system.
2. The combined treatment of selective adsorption and subsequent IgG may be superior to other treatment regimes, since the removal of the postulated circulating humoral agent prior to IgG infusion may allow for a more effective immunomodulation, as the humoral agent will not interfere with IgG after removal.

The validity of those hypotheses can be tested only in a large series, preferably in a multicenter study.

We propose the following three treatment arms:
1. Selective adsorption using a TR 350 column.
2. Selective adsorption using a TR 350 column and subsequent administration of intravenous immunoglobulin G.
3. Intravenous immunoglobulin G alone.

92

A two lumen catheter-system for investigation of spinal fluid dynamics and lumbar long-term pressure recording

Jost V, Stoll M, Hamann G, Schimrigk K
Department of Neurology, University of Saarland, FRG

Measurement of outflow resistance and compliance of the cerebrospinal fluid system according to Marmarou (2) and Kosteljanetz (1) are essential in diagnosis of normal pressure hydrocephalus and in deciding about an OP-indication. Further a long-term recording of intracranial pressure and szintigraphy of the spinal fluid compartement is important. Implementing this measurement, which requires application of bolus and constant steady state infusion of physiological NaCl-solution into the cerebrospinal fluid system, combined with simultaneous pressure recording, some methodological problems arise. A common one lumen catheter is not suitable for correct registration of the important peak-pressure while applying the bolus of NaCl solution. But using a second lumbar puncture for volume application stresses the patient considerably. Besides artefacts caused by movements of the patient are increased using this method. Up to now a double lumen catheter for this purpose is not tested.

We used a two lumen catheter, usually employed as cava catheter for neonates (18 Ga), which was lumbarly inserted through a 14 Ga tubule. Pressure measurement and registration were done using a Statham-pressure transducer and a Siemens Sirecust 404 monitor, connected to a personal computer (PC) by an analog-digital conversion card. The PC software was developed by us not only for this purpose and is described in other places. The results using this catheter were similiar to those obtained using two lumbar punctures and showed significantly less artefacts. Further the installation of a long-term pressure measurement was possible. The resistance to outflow values obtained up to know were normal (<12 mmHg/ml/min) in all patients. The long-term pressure recordings showed no pathological wave-forms. An important advantage of this method was the application in comfortable supine position and the restriction to a single lumbar puncture. So a practicable method, which provides an easy handling, less inconvenience for the patient and low costs is introduced.

1. Kosteljanetz M (1985) Resistance to outflow of cerebrospinal fluid determined by bolus injection technique and constant rate steady state infusion in humans. Neurosurgery 16: 336-340.
2. Marmarou A, Shulman K, La Morgese J (1975) Compartmental analysis of compliance and outflow resistance of the cerebrospinal fluid system. J Neurosurg. 43: 523-534.

93

PC- Based Monitoring of Intracraniell Pressure

Stoll M, Hamann G, Jost V, Schimrigk K
Departemnt of Neurology, University of Saarland, FRG

By managing neurological intensive care patients with intracranial pressure (ICP) rise, the measurement and recording of ICP and simultaneously of arterial blood pressure, is of special interest. Therapy of brain edema and hypertension can be controlled using these parameters. ICP measurement is also important in the diagnosis of the various subtypes of hydrocephalus. For this purpose we developed an inexpensive and easy installed system, comprising a PC and a conventional monitor (Siemens Sirecust 404) connected by an Analog-Digital conversion card. Gaeltec epidural transducers were used for pressure measurement. The software specially developed for this system stores, demonstrates and prints the online-course and the trend. Further it is possible to view the online course of conspicuous parts of the trend retrospectively and to use these values for statistical analysis. Object-orientated software development techniques were used for flexible output on screen, printer or picture file.

In a pilot study we examined 5 patients (pat) suffering from intracerebral hemorrhage, 2 pat with subarachnoid haemorrhage, 1 pat with cerebellar infarction and 1 pat with cerebellar abscesses. ICP measurement was performed for 3 to 10 days. Based on the individual requirements it was possible to reduce the dose of hyperosmolar drugs by 80% when compared with a standardized therapy protocoll. Besides it was possible to recognize dangerous pressure rises in time. Further we examined intracranial pressure dynamic in 6 patients conspicious of normal pressure hydrocephalus by measurement of compliance, pressure volume index and resistance to outflow (2) using a bolus injection technique and a constant rate steady state infusion (1). Additionally a 24 h long-term pressure recording was done in each patient. In these cases pressure measurement and simultaneous application of physiologic NaCl-solution were performed employing both lumens of a lumbar 2-lumen catheter.

Our investigation shows the possibility to recognize dangerous intracraniell pressure rises and to optimize brain edema therapy by ICP-monitoring. By using the described system it was possible to treat dangerous pressure rises in time and save a considerable amount of hyperosmolar drugs. The use in clinical routine was enforced by easy handling and low costs compared with other commercial alternatives.

1. Kosteljanetz M (1985) Resistance to outflow of cerebrospinal fluid determined by bolus injection technique and constant rate steady state infusion in humans. Neurosurgery 16: 336-340.

2. Marmarou A, Shulman K, La Morgese J (1975) Compartmental analysis of compliance and outflow resistance of the cerebrospinal fluid system. J Neurosurg. 43: 523-534.

94

Etiology, diagnosis and treatment of syringomyelia

Donauer E and Steudel WI:
Neurosurgical Clinic of the Saarland University
Homburg/Saar Germany

As manifold as the terminology of syringomyelia are the hypotheses of the etiology. These are extremely diverse and it is necessary to know as much as possible about its causes in each individual case before treatment or therapy can be initiated. Fortunately nowadays with MRI without and with gadolinium it is possible to diagnose intramedullar cavities safely in patients. In addition to the high quality of the morphological documentation, the MR especially the cine-MR provides information on pathophysiological details of the flow and intracavitary pressure dependant pulsations of the CSF.

The findings from our own experimental studies on cats (n=68) are surprisingly similar to those from MR in humans (n=62). The term syringomyelia is only used for dysraphic cavities in the medulla.

In cases without any sign of a malformation, for example Chiari malformation or basilar impression, special attention must be given of intraspinal tumors or other cystic intramedullar lesions as cause of cysts in the spinal cord.

Animal models have enabled us to study a form of syringomyelia which very closely resembles that brought about by dysraphic malformations in the human being and to examine the effectiveness of certain types of surgical therapy.

We could differentiate three types of the so-called hydro- or syringomyelia.

1: The so-called hydromyelia, or syringobulbia, corresponds to experimental closure of the foramina Luschkae with cotton swabs, with continuous dilation of the cavity along the total spinal cord canal especially into the cervicomedullary transition.

2: The hydromyelia is known from very deep sitting tonsils of the cerebellum (Arnold-Chiari 2) with a narrow central canal in craniocervical transition and the balloon-like dilation of the syrinx under the narrowness corresponds to our experimnetal type of well-known kaolin hydrocephalus with a broad kaolin cuff in the craniocervical subarachnoid space.

3: In hydromyelia as seen in Arnold-Chiari 1 or patients with scars in craniocervical transition with a narrow canal in the region of the first body of the cervical spine a more slightly dilation of the central canal is observed by mild injection of kaolin in the cisterna magna.

The experimental studies confirm observations that 3 types of syringomyelia in patients depending of the type of CSF circulation disturbances.

The strongly development of cavities along the dorsal raphe in our experiments were similar to what was thought to be characteristic of processes involved in neurochisis (Padget 1970). The partial pressure compensation between inner and outer spinal and cerebral CSF spaces is responsible for the complete dilation of the central canal. This and the CSF outflow from the filum terminale can compensate the increased base pressure. But acute pressure changes like in breathing, coughing or venous pressure changes cannot be sufficiently be compensated. Intraventriculary injected contrast medium or dye show a diffuse flow of CSF from the filum terminale into the spinal subarachnoid space. Morphologically there are no channels. Our experiments show that not the reduction of CSF capacity and not the separation of the dilated central canal are responsible for the progression of syringomyelia. The important point is the reduction of the possibilities for fast compensation of pressure changes caused by the obstruction of the outlets of the fourth ventricle. The dilated central canal is a natural shunt, but this is not sufficient. The drain is considerably prolonged and has increased flow resistance. In the filum terminale there is an outflow of CSF but not an open end of the central canal. So only parts of the CSF pressure can be compensated, and only with delay. This demonstrates also the necessity of an early surgical intervention by the human progressive syringomyelia. As first step we recommend the decompression of the craniocervical transition and as second operative approach the syringoarachnoid shunting in cases of large intraspinal cavities.

95

THE INFLUENCE OF SLOW-RELEASE THEOPHYLLINE ON NOCTURNAL OXYGEN SATURATION AND SLEEP ARCHITECTURE IN SLEEP-APNEA SYNDROME.

J.M. Elek, Th. Orfgen, J.P. Sieb & R. Dengler, Department of Neurology, University of Bonn, FRG.

Theophylline is used in the therapy of sleep-apnea syndrome (SAS). On one hand it is reported to reduce the occurrence of nocturnal apneas, on the other hand it may also considerably reduce sleep quality. We investigated the influence of slow-release theophylline on nocturnal oxygen saturation (SaO_2), thus monitoring the effects of both apneas and hypopneas, and on sleep architecture in 10 patients with sleep-apnea syndrome (mean age 55 years, mean apnea-index 27/h). Polysomnographic recordings were carried out without and under medication with slow-release theophylline (interval between recordings 3-4 nights, evening dose of 6 mg/kg body weight). Overall, the SaO_2-profile under medication showed a nonsignificant trend towards a higher percentage of hypoxia time of total sleep time. Individual reactions to theophylline, however, were considerably variable: 30% of the patients showed normal nocturnal SaO_2-profiles under medication, 30% remained unchanged, 40% deteriorated somewhat with respect to their SaO_2-situation. 60% of the patients reported subjective improvement of daytime sleepiness. Sleep-stage-analyses revealed a significant (p < 0.005) reduction of sleep-efficiency with longer waking times during the sleep period and earlier awakening in the morning under theophylline. Subjectively 30% of patients complained about a reduced sleep quality. In summary, the effect of slow-release theophylline on the nocturnal SaO_2-profile in patients with SAS is variable, possible responders can only be identified by trial and error. We observed a significant reduction of sleep-efficiency under theophylline, which in about one third of the patients became clinically relevant.

96

Control of the therapy of intracranial pressure by means of daily excretion of meta- and normetanephrines in urine in patients with intracerebral haemorrhage

Hamann G. , Strittmatter M., Holzer G., Haaß A., Schimrigk K.

Department of Neurology, University of the Saarland, D-6650 Homburg/Saar

Introduction: One of the typical complications after spontaneous intracerebral haemorrhages (ICH) is the disturbance of the intracranial pressure (ICP) with especially dangerous rises of ICP. These ICP-elevations can be accompanied by sympathicotonic deregulation with rises of the catecholamines in plasma. Thus, the urine-metabolites are elevated, especially the metanephrines (MN) and the normetanephrines (NMN). Aim of this study is the presentation of the therapeutical effects in these hormones.

Patients and Methods: 18 patients with acute spontaneous ICH participated in this study. There were 11 male and 7 female, 3 patients with haemorrhage of the pons, 1 of the cerebellum and 14 patients with typically haemorrhages of the capsula interna and the basal ganglia. Mean age was 61,5 +/- 13,7 years. ICP-rises were treated with hyperosmolaric agents, especially glycerol (oral) and sorbitol (intravenously). Elevation of head and hyperventilation were part of the basic therapy.

The urines of the patients were collected over 24 h every day. The first 21 days after the initial haemorrhages MN and NMN were determined daily by means of a HPLC with electrochemical detection.

Results: 9 out of 18 patients showed an inconspicuous clinical time course after the ICH without any severe complication (group 1). ICP-rises were rare and therapy of these rises was always sufficient. The other 9 patients developed severe complications and frequent ICP-rises with dangerous clinical detoriations like beginning transtentorial herniation (group 2). 7 out of 9 patients of group 1 showed no elevation of the MN or NMN over the time course, only 2 patients had slight elevated MN and NMN. Whereas 7 out of 9 patients of group 2 produced intensive elevations of NMN and/or MN. The 10-fold of normal values were seen. Only 2 patients of group 2 had no disturbances of the MN/NMN.

These differences were significant (X^2 = 5,55, p< 0,01) using the X^2-test. Glasgow Coma Outcome Scale reached 2,66 in mean of the group 1 and 4,44 in group 2. This statistically difference was confirmed by 5 death in group 2, whereas only 2 patients of group 1 died.

Discussion: Normal MN and NMN were accompanied by good clinical course, good outcome and especially a sufficient therapy of the ICP-rises. Whereas elevated NMN/MN were joined with a severe and complicated clinical course and reduced effect of the hyperosmolaric therapy. The prognostic relevance of MN/NMN-elevations could be confirmed. The urine-catecholamines are potent indicators of a sufficient therapy and allow controlling of the management of patients with elevated ICP.

97

The Paresis Score - a new instrument for the prospective dokumentation of the clinical course in 30 patients with Guillain-Barré syndrome and CIDP

F. Rosenow, W.F. Haupt, A. Rose, H. Borberg*

Klinik und Poliklinik für Neurologie und Psychiatrie - Neurologie and (*) Klinik I für Innere Medizin der Universität zu Köln, Joseph-Stelzmann Str. 9, 5000 Köln 41, Federal Republic of Germany

Introduction: The Guillain-Barré syndrom is nowadays the most common acute and life threatening disease of the peripheral nervous system. Even though the prognosis is generally good up to 5% of (often young) patients die from complications. Plasma exchange [1] and recently the intravenous application of 7S-immunoglobulins [2] have been shown to be effective therapies in two multicenter studies. In these studies a functional score (F-score, 0=healthy to 5=ventilated and 6=dead) originally published by Hughes et al.[3] and a sum of the MRC-scores of 2x6 muscle groups (MRC-score; 0=panparalysis to 60=full strength) were used to follow the clinical course and for definition of end points. Both scores were shown to be have a high interobserver agreement [4]. An F-score of 4 or 5 corresponds with a wide range of MRC-scores [4], which demonstrates the value of a more defined score for documentation of the clinical status. Both scores do not include prognostically important parameters like vital capacity and cranial nerve involvement.

Methods: Since 1989, the **Paresis Score** (P-score, 0=healthy to 100=panparalysis) developed in Cologne has been used in the prospective follow up of GBS- and CIDP-patients. This score includes the F- and MRC-scores for their proven reliability and value as well as to make results comparable. Subscores for vital capacity and cranial nerve involvement are included for their obvious clinical importance. Measurements of grip strength (by the "My Gripper", 0-55 kp) were taken into account since they were shown to correlate with the CMAP of the abductor pollicis brevis (APB) in patients with CIDP [5] and because these CMAPs are the prognostically most valuable electrophysiological parameter in GBS-patients [6].

Results: The **Paresis Score** has been used 290 times in 30 GBS-patients. Patients were followed for up to two years. Depending on the degree of paresis and the patients´ ability to cooperate one examination takes 10 to 25 minutes. In only 8 of 290 examinations the patients self-assessment did not correspond with the course shown by the **Paresis Score**. Even small changes in the clinical status like the intermittent "relapses" seen after immunoglobulin or plasma therapy were registered. Graphic correlations of the P-score and of grip strength with the APB-CMAPs can be demonstrated. The median of the APB-CMAP in 24 normal controls was 12.5 mV. If the APB-CMAP was >11mV in GBS-patients, the **Paresis Score** was never higher than 18. If the P-score was over 45 CMAPs were higher than 5 (but less than 10) in only 2 cases. If grip strength was less than 15 kp the CMAPs never exceeded 11mV. On the other hand: if grip strength was over 28 kp, CMAPs were less than 10 in only 4 patients.

References

1. The Guillain-Barré Syndrome Study group (1985) Plasmapheresis and acute Guillain-Barré syndrome. Neurology 35 :1096-1104
2. van der Meché FGA, Schmitz PIM, The Dutch Guillain-Barré Study Group (1992) A randomized trial comparing intravenous immune globulin and plasma exchange in Guillain-Barré syndrome. NEJM 326 :1123-1129
3. Hughes R, Newsom-Davis J, Perkin G, Pierce J (1978) Controlled trial of prednisolone in acute polyneuropathy. Lancet 2 :750-753
4. Kleyweg RP, van der Meché FGA, Schmitz PIM (1991) Interobserver agreement in the assessment of muscle strength and functional abilities in Guillain-Barré syndrome. Muscle & Nerve 14 : 1103-1109
5. van der Meché FGA, Vermeulen M, Busch HFM (1989) Chronic inflammatory demyelinating polyneuropathy - conduction failure before and during immunoglobulin or plasma therapy. Brain 112 : 1563-1571
6. McKhann GM (1990) Guillain-Barré syndrome : Clinical and therapeutic Observations. Ann Neurol 27(suppl) : 13-16

98

SEROLOGICAL PARAMETERS IN SPORADIC AMYOTROPHIC LATERALS SCLEROSIS

Westarp ME, Flügel RM, Bartmann P, Fuchs D, Hoff-Jörgensen R, Clausen D, Westarp MP, Kornhuber HH

Treating 45 individuals with adult idiopathic ALS (lower and upper motor neuron involvement without multifocal conduction block or IgM or relevant IgG anti-ganglioside antibodies), we observed elevated circulating immune complexes in 11/27, and 13/14 neurological sera from 1988 to 1991 who had >50 mg/L immune complexes indeed associated with motor neuron disease (6/27 ALS patients versus 1/79 control patients with suspected collagenoses). Excluding patients with abnormal total serum IgG, immunoglobulin isotype IgG_3 was decreased below 0.4 mg/L in 20/24 (mean 0.29 g/l $\pm$ .02 SEM). 13/32 ALS patients had enzyme-linked sorbent assay (ELISA) serum antibodies against human spuma retrovirus (HSRV) envelope and/or gag.capsid antigens, so far confirmed by specific immunoblots in seven patients (p<0.01 compared to regional and neurological controls). 25/920 German surgical patients had been tested HSRV seropositive before (Mahnke 1992). Six male HSRV-positive patients only reacted to either HSRV-gag or HSRV-env, none of them had simultaneously elevated immune complexes. 28 ALS sera have at present been tested in a blocking ELISA using maedi-visna virus antigen (competition with specific antibodies relative to human control sera); ALS sera reduced specific binding better than 22 sera from matched patient controls (mean ELISA optical density reduced by 11.0% $\pm$ 1.9 (ALS) versus 6.9% $\pm$ 1.0 (patient controls), p<0.05).

Despite reports on unchanged mean serum immunoglobulins in ALS (Chancellor AM et.al 1992), we found quantitatively abnormal concentrations of IgG, IgM and/or IgA in 14/32 patients (references: IgG 800 - 1600, IgA 90 - 450, IgM (f) 60 - 250 and (m) 70 - 280 mg/dl). Serum β_2-microglobulin concentrations were normal in the CSF of 6 and in 45 sera of 32 patients. CA-19-9, a marker for chronic gastrointestinal inflammation, was elevated (to 16.1, 18, 35, 45 and 1118 U/l, healthy reference <14 U/l) in 5/12 ALS patients examined; malignant alterations were excluded.

In lack of more efficient options, we treated eleven (HIV-negative) ALS patients with 500 mg/d zidovudine (Retrovir^R) p.o. over 2-10 months. In 8/9 compliant patients we observed a reduction of serum creatine kinase two days to two weeks after begin of medication, while physical activities remained unchanged and zidovudine given to non-ALS patients rather increased serum CK. In 3/4 zidovudine patients, circulating immune complexes fell upon medication, in one patient from 96 mg/l to <2.5 mg/l. No signs or symptoms for a drug-induced mitochondrial myopathy were observed. One patient reported less frequent fasciculations after onset of zidovudine therapy, and one patient reported a transient stabilisation (holding of razor). Pre-therapeutic rates of progression had not been available to assess clinical effects more reliably. ALS leaves its marks outside the neuro-muscular system, and some of these serological parameters may respond to antiretroviral therapy.

Dr.M.E.Westarp, D-79 Ulm University Dept. Neurology Psychiatrisches Landeskrankenhaus D-7942 Zwiefalten

99

SLOWER PROGRESSION OF AMYOTROPHIC LATERAL SCLEROSIS (ALS) FOLLOWING INTRATHECALLY-ADMINISTERED NATURAL FIBROBLAST INTERFERON-BETA (IFN-BETA)

Westphal K.P., Bauer J., Laupheimer H., Westarp M.E., Hülser P., Schreiber H., Baumgärtner K., Wollinsky K.H., van Eick H.*, Kornhuber H.H.
Dept. Neurology, RKU, Oberer Eselsberg 45, D- 7900 Ulm
*Rentschler GmbH, D-7958 Laupheim, Germany

Based on the hypothesis that ALS is of viral etiology (Jolicoeur et al. 1991, Westarp et al. 1992) a therapeutic trial with the antiviral human fibroblast interferon-beta was carried out. In 17 patients with a proved diagnosis of ALS, clinical investigations were carried out during and following 6 months of intrathecally applied IFN-beta (total dose of 18x1 Mio.E). During the first four weeks, patients received IFN-beta (1 Mio.E) twice a week and during the following 5 months twice per month. Every 4-6 weeks, patients were independently rated by a neurologist and an experienced physiotherapist for muscle force, signs of atrophy and spasticity of the upper and lower extremities. Furthermore, patients were assessed by the Norris ALS score. 6 of the 17 patients interrupted the treatment for various reasons. Of the remaining 11 patients, 7 based on the Norris scale, 5 on the physiotherapist's investigations and 8 on the neurologist's investigations revealed during the 6 months of IFN-beta treatment, a slower disease progression than in the 6 months following the end of IFN-beta treatment. An unchanged progression during and after the IFN-beta therapy was revealed by the Norris scale in 3 cases, by the physiotherapist's evaluations in 5 cases and by the neurologist's investigations in 3 cases. A faster progression during treatment compared to 6 months after treatment was seen in 1 patient (Norris scale and physiotherapist). An analysis of the score values as between the physiotherapist and the neurologist revealed a correlation coefficient of 0.74102; $p = 0.0001$ (Pearson Coefficient of Correlation).

After the end of therapy, patients rated subjective side-effects on a self-rating scale with values between 0 (no side-effects) and 10 (severe side-effects). The highest mean values were obtained for feelings of exhaustion (3.7) and for lack of appetite (3.7) followed by pain of limbs (3.3). No exhaustion was recorded in 1 out of 15 patients, no limb pains in 5, no lack of appetite in 6 and no back pain in 7 out of 15 patients.

Highest drug fever was measured after the first intrathecal application with a median of 38.6°C; drug fever decreased during the following applications combined with a decreased dose of paracetamol. The median of paracetamol dose in the first application was 1400 mg, in the second application 1000 mg, in the third application 900 mg, and then a relatively constant dose between 500-700 mg. With this dosage, drug fever was below 38°C (median) during the course of the various applications.

Drug fever higher than 40°C, leucopenia, thrombocytopenia, an increase of PTT, and a decrease of fibrinogen, as observed during intravenous therapy were not observed during our investigation using intrathecally-applied interferon-beta.

The results perhaps suggest that intrathecally-administered IFNbeta may have a positive effect on the progression of amyotrophic lateral sclerosis.

References

1. Jolicoeur P, Rassart E, DesGroseillersL, Robitaille Y, Paquette Y, Kay DG: Retrovirus-induced motor neuron disease of mice: molecular basis of neurotropism and paralysis. Adv Neurol 56: 481-493, 1991.

2. Westarp ME, Westphal KP, Kolde G, Wollinsky KH, Westarp MP, Dickob M, Kornhuber HH: Dermal, serological and CSF changes in amyotrophic lateral sclerosis with and without intrathecal interferon beta treatment. Int J Clin Pharmacol Ther Toxicol 30: 81-93, 1992.

100

Cyclophosphamide treatment in disorders of the peripheral motoneuron: clinical response in correlation to anti-GM1 serum antibody titre

F. Heidenreich, L. Leifeld and R. Benecke
Department of Neurology, Heinrich-Heine University
Moorenstraße 5, 4000 Düsseldorf, Germany

Increased titres of antibodies to gangliosides, in particular to GM1 (anti-GM1), are detectable in the serum of patients with multifocal motor neuropathy with conduction block (MMN) and acquired lower motor neuron syndroms (LMN). They are mostly polyclonal IgM antibodies, but M-proteins with specificity for GM1 and less commonly also increased titres of IgG anti-GM1 have been found. Although the pathogenetic significance of anti-GM1 is not yet clarified they point to an underlying immune process in these disorders and this is supported by their frequent association with the acute Guillain-Barré syndrome (GBS), an immune-mediated demyelinating neuropathy. Patients with MMN and LMN were often misdiagnosed as degenerative motor neuron disorder e.g. as beginning amyotrophic lateral sclerosis (ALS). Increased serum anti-GM1 may be taken as a justification for an immunosuppressive treatment. In a number of cases a favourable outcome after treatment with cyclophosphamide has been reported while corticosteroids and other immunosuppressants were not effective (Feldman et al. Ann Neurol (1991) 30:397-401). However, systematic studies of the therapeutic response are not available.

We determined serum anti-GM1 in patients with motor neuropathies including MMN and with pure LMN in comparison to ALS, chronic inflammatory demyelinating neuropathy (CIDP), paraproteinemic neuropathy, myasthenia gravis and normal controls by a modified ELISA. Serum titres of IgM anti-GM1 increased by more than 3 SD above the mean of 35 controls were found in 3 of 5 patients with MMN and 3 of 12 with LMN and also in 3 of 29 patients with CIDP and in 11 of 36 patients with GBS. One patient with MMN had increased serum IgG antibodies to GM1. In an ongoing study three patients with MMN and three with LMN were treated with cyclophosphamide at oral doses of 2 - 3 mg per kg bodyweight per day for a period of 12 - 24 months while performing intensive physiotherapy. Blood cell counts were initially checked at weekly intervals, later twice a month and the dose adjusted to a leukocyte count of 3 - 4000 /ul with 600-1000 lymphocytes/ul. Neurological follow-up examinations including electrophysiological testing and determination of serum anti-GM1 titres were done every 2 - 3 months. The clinical response was assessed by a score derived from manual muscle force testing and grading by the MRC scale. The treatment was generally tolerated without side-effects. All three patients with MMN improved considerably in terms of their muscle force and two of them returned to normal life with unaffected use of hands and feet. Improvement began 6 - 9 months after initiation of treatment and continued over the following 6 - 12 months. It was accompanied by a normalization of the clinical score and a decrease of anti-GM1 serum titres to normal values. Electrophysiological testing revealed persistent motor conduction block in all three patients. In one patient the treatment was finished after 16 months without clinical relapse or increase of anti-GM1 serum titre up to now. In the three LMN patients one patient with predominantly distal affection showed a comparable improvement. In a further patient with LMN and predominantly proximal paresis the disease has continued to progress inspite of effective immunosuppression over one year. In the third LMN patient the clinical status remained unchanged. Oral cyclophosphamide treatment of MMN appears to be effective and safe. In this disorder the anti-GM1 serum titre is of diagnostic value and may be used as a marker to monitor treatment response. In LMN the role of immunosuppressiion and anti-GM1 is not clear, but the number of LMN patients studied is too small to permit final conclusions.

101

Constipation in PD - Diagnosis and Therapy

Wolfgang H. Jost and Klaus Schimrigk

Dep. of Neurology at the University of Saarland,

Homburg / Saar, Germany

Besides the triad of akinesia, rigor and tremor, the most frequently recorded symptoms in Parkinson's disease (PD) are due to autonomic dysfunction. The diagnosis of cardiovascular autonomic disturbance is well researched and is, in many places, used as a part of the routine diagnostic work-up. Investigating the function of the gastrointestinal tract is more costly, and less well tolerated by the patient; hence it is less common use as a diagnostic method. By modifying a well known protocol (1) we have investigated the oro-anal transit time (2). Over 6 days, each day the patients took a gelatine capsule containing 10 radio-opaque pellets. On the seventh day a plain abdominal x-ray was taken. The number of pellets seen on the x-ray divided by ten gave the transit time, in days. Through this investigation we found that 80% of our 20 patients with idiopathic PD had a prolonged transit time (2). Patients taking anticholinergic drugs were excluded due to the constipating effect of these drugs. Taking the hypothesis that the cause of the slowing was beside a central disturbance the degeneration of the myenteric plexus, we treated the patients with 5 mg of cisapride, twice daily. This drug causes a selective increase in the acetylcholine output of the myenteric plexus.

We investigated 25 patients, with sex- and age matched controls. Their average age was 68.5 years. The patients had an average disability score of 17 on the Webster scale (3). None of the patients were bed-ridden, none gave a history of having had an abdominal operation or gastro-intestinal disease. Their anti-Parkinsonian medication (up to three of: L-DOPA + BENSERAZIDE; SELEGILINE; BROMOCRIPTINE; LISURIDE) was not altered throughout the trial period.

In the group of PD patients, 20 of the 25 showed a prolonged transit time. In the control group one patient showed a delay in transit, with two others on the borderline of normality. The average pellet count in the PD group was 47.4 pellets. In the 20 of these showing delayed transit the count was 53.8 pellets. In the control group the average pellet count was 22.9 pellets.

The patients with prolonged transit time (10 male, 10 female, average age 68,3 years) subsequently received 5 mg of cisapride, twice daily. The trial regime was repeated in these patients, and after a week the new x-ray revealed a lower number of pellets in every patient. The average count had fallen from 53.8 in the first film, to 30.4 when repeated while taking cisapride. No difference between sexes was seen. No adverse effects were observed during the week of cisapride therapy.

These observations show that cisapride seems to be a useful therapy for the constipation often seen in PD. Whether these results would be replicated in a larger group of patients needs to be assessed in a prospective, double-blind, cross-over, multi-centre study. Further studies would show whether this effect continues with long-term therapy.

1) Hinton JM, Lennard-Jones JE, Young AC (1969) A new method for studying gut transit times using radioopaque markers. Gut 10: 842-847

2) Jost WH, Schimrigk K (1991) Constipation in Parkinson's disease. Klin Wochenschr 69: 906-909

3) Webster DD (1968) Critical analysis of the disability in Parkinson's disease. Modern treatment 5: 257-282

102

L-DOPA SLOW-RELEASE VERSUS L-DOPA STANDARD: PHARMACOKINETIC AND MOTOR RESPONSE IN PARKINSONIAN PATIENTS WITH AND WITHOUT FLUCTUATIONS

N. Bergemann[1], H. Baas[1], L. Demisch[2] & P.-A. Fischer[1]

[1]Dept. of Neurology, [2]Dept. of Psychiatry

University of Frankfurt/Main, Germany

For the therapeutic management of fluctuations in long-term therapy of Parkinsonian patients L-dopa slow-release preparations might be an alternative therapy strategy even if some of the results are discussed controversially. Pharmacokinetic and pharmacodynamic studies provide evidence of an adequate galenic as the slow-release principle. This serves as a rational basis for a possible clinical benefit in patients with fluctuations.

Under the condition of a single dose pharmacokinetic this study investigates the pharmacological behavior and motor response of a new L-dopa slow-release formulation in comparison to L-dopa standard in Parkinsonian patients with and without fluctuations. Therefore, a controlled, randomized, double-blind 4-time cross-over study was carried out in twelve Parkinsonian patients with fluctuations (7 men, 5 women; mean age 60.3 ($\pm$10.4) years; range: 41-79 years) and twelve patients without fluctuations (6 men, 6 women; mean age 61.5 ($\pm$8.8) years; range 49-80 years). The mean duration of disease was 11.5 ($\pm$5.1) years in patients with, and 3.5 ($\pm$8.2) years in patients without fluctuations. In the group with fluctuations, 1 of the patients was stage II, 4 were stage III, and 7 stage IV of Hoehn and Yahr's classification; in the group without fluctuations, 7 patients were stage II, 4 stage III, and 1 patient was stage IV. Three different doses (125 mg, 225 mg, 375 mg) of the newly formulated L-dopa/benserazide slow-release preparation (ASTA H995) or L-dopa/ benserazide standard respectively were administered on four different days within a total of ten days. The patients had no other Parkinsonian medication during the study days except Selegiline. On each study day L-dopa serum-concentration was determined every 15 minutes over a period of 6 hours; in parallel, motor response was rated continuously using the Columbia University Rating Scale and the patients carried out the Purdue Pegboard as well as a modification of the Webster Step Second Test.

Preliminary results show no significant difference in the pharmacokinetic behavior in patients with versus without fluctuations. Altogether, the results correspond to the predicted pharmacokinetic curves in the sense of different C_{max}, T_{max} and AUC of L-dopa standard and the diverse L-dopa slow-release preparations: The L-dopa standard curves show the well-known peak, the slow-release formulations cause a delayed increase of L-dopa plasma concentration without a clear peak which was maintained for a prolonged period of time; the different slow-release doses correspond to the different C_{max}-values, the duration of motor effect of a single dose of L-dopa slow-release was substantially longer than L-dopa standard. The minimal effective L-dopa plasma concentration of 0.8 mg/ml occurs in all patients except one with L-dopa standard and in all with slow-release 375 mg L-dopa/benserazide, in most of the patients (14 out of 23) with 250 mg, but only in 4 out of 23 patients with 125 mg slow-release L-dopa/benserazide formulation.

With regard to inter-individual differences the conditions of unsatisfactory L-dopa response are to be determined and the development of individual therapy strategies under short-term drug monitoring of L-dopa medication is necessary.

103

THE CHRONIC STIMULATION OF THE NUCLEUS VENTRALIS INTERMEDIUS THALAMI IN THE TREATMENT OF PARKINSONIAN TREMOR.

F. Alesch°, E.Fertl*, E.Auff*, W.Koos°

°Neurochirurgische Univ.Klinik, *Neurologische Univ.Klinik
Währinger Gürtel 18-20, A-1090 Vienna, Austria

Based on the observation that low-frequency (50 Hz) electric stimulation of the ventral intermediate thalamic nucleus (VIM) increases parkinsonian tremor, while higher frequencies (>100 Hz) lead to suppression of the tremor, we implanted in 10 patients into 12 thalami (2 bilateral) under stereotactic conditions a stimulation electrode and connected it subcutaneusly to an implanted Neurostimulator (ITREL II, MEDTRONIC). Stimulation brought complete suppression of tremor in 8 cases, major improvement in 1 and minor in 1. There was no significant effect on any other existing symptoms of Parkinson's disease. Follow-up ranges from 2 to 28 months. No complications or escape phenomena have been observed so far. We consider this procedure as an effective and safe alternative to conventional thalamotomy. Unlike the latter it is a non-ablative procedure. So adverse side effects such as dystonia, eye movement disorders, speech disorders or even hemiparesis can be ruled out. It should be considered in cases in which drug therapy has failed to affect parkinsonian tremor.

104

LONG-TERM SURVIVORS WITH NEUROEPITHELIAL BRAIN TUMORS - NEUROLOGICAL FINDINGS, CT AND PSYCHOLOGICAL RESULTS

B. Bauer, B. Schmidt, G. Grau, S. Henschel
Department of Neurology, Hospital for Nervous Diseases,
University of Rostock

The progress in diagnostic procedures and treatment has prolonged the survival time of patients with gliomatous brain tumors (1,2). We have treated 107 patients with neuroepithelial tumors postoperativily by radiotherapy (grade 2; n=23) or by combined radio- and chemotherapy (grade 3 and 4; n=84). Up to now 22 (20,6%) of these patients have survived more than 5 years (grade2: n=9, grade 3: n=8, grade 4: n=5). The histological diagnoses were: 16 astrocytomas (72,7%), 3 glioblastomas, 1 ependymoma, 1 oligodendroglioma and 1 sarcoma. The surgical procedure was a subtotal resection in 17 cases (77%) and a total resection in 5 patients according to the neurosurgeons' description. 1 patient was reoperated on at recurrence, 2 patients were operated 3 times. All patients were treated postoperatively by limited-volume irradiation (57-60 Gy). Patients with 3rd and 4th grade tumors received additional chemotherapy every 8 weeks for 2 years (1). The average age of long-term survivors was 29,8 + 9,6 years at onset of disease. Only 4/22 (18,2%) of long-term survivors were older than 40 years, but 8/107 (63,6%) of all treated patients had an age of >40 years. The time period between first symptoms of disease and operation was longer than 1 year in 50% with the longest time of 15,3 years. 19/22 (86,4%) of long-term survivors had epileptic seizures, but only 35/107 (32,7%) of all patients had this symptom. The group of long-term survivors revealed an accumulation of prognostically favourable factors such as young age at onset of disease, long case history, frequent history of epileptic seizures and low grade tumors.

The long-term survivors were reinvestigated 6,9 + 1,9 years after operation by neurological examination, CT-scan, and assessment of intellectual functions and subjective well-being. 8 patients had neurological deficits (hemiparesis, aphasia, ataxia or brain organic syndrome), whereas 14 patients had normal neurological findings. The Karnofsky-scores were 89,5 + 13,6 points (range: 70 - 100). The majority of patients reported a good subjective well-being as proven by different questionnaires (4). The total score of cognitive functions (verbal intelligence, reasoning, concentration, speed, memory and learning) was in the lower range of standard (x = 7,85 + 2,39 points, standard: 10 + 3 points). The highest reduction was found in tests checking the complex cognitive functions. 16/22 long-term survivors have also been investigated for their cognitive functions 1,2 + 0,6 years post operation. The results of the total cognitive score did not differ significantly from the actual values (8,46 + 2,45 versus 8,19 + 2.44 points, t = 1,30, corr. 0,94). In contrast to reports of the literature (2,3) only 1 patient became demented. This fact may mainly be due to avoidance of whole brain irradiation in our concept of treatment.

20 actual CT-scans did not show any signs of recurrence. Only in 2 cases a small tumor residue was seen by CT. With regard to long-term consequences of irradiation and chemotherapy we found 11 patients (group 1) without signs of leukencephalopathy, 7 patients (group 2) with negligible and 4 patients (group 3) with moderate or severe leukencephalopathy. The corresponding total cognitive scores were significantly different between the groups (group 1: 8,9 + 2,7, group 2: 6,6 + 1,0, group 3: 5,4 + 2,7: 1 vs 2 t=2,16, p<0,05; 1 vs 3 t=2,25, p<0,05; 2 vs 3 not significant).
If CT-results were analysed with regard to enlargement of arachnoidal spaces and/or ventricular system, 9 patients (group I) showed no signs of enlargement, 5 patients (group II) showed enlargement of one system and in 8 patients (group III) both systems were enlarged. The total score of cognitive functions was 9,29 + 2,82 in group I, 7,06 + 1,50 in group II and 6,02 + 1,92 in group III (I vs III t=2,76, p<0,05). The strongest intellectual impairments were found in patients with combination of leukencepha- lopathy and enlargement of subarachnoidal spaces and/or ventricular system. In most cases there was a good correla- tion between morphological changes in CT and intellectual functions.

1. Bauer B (1990) Psychiat Neurol Med Psychol 42: 485-493
2. Imperato JP, Paleogolos NA, Vick NA (1991) Ann Neurol 28: 818-822
3. Garden AS, Maor MH, Yung WKA, Bruner JM, Woo SY, Moser RP, Lee Y-Y (1991) Radiother Oncol 20: 99-110
4. Schmidt B, Bauer B (1986) Psychiat Neurol Med Psychol 38: 584 - 591

105

RATIONAL DIAGNOSTIC STRATEGY IN SPORADIC PRIMARY CEREBRAL MALIGNANT LYMPHOMAS

Dieter F. Braus, Karl Schwechheimer, Benedikt Volk
Department of Neuropathology, Institute of Pathology,
Albert-Ludwigs-University of Freiburg; Germany

Primary cerebral malignant Non-Hodgkin`s lymphoma (PCML) is a rare tumour, but it is occurring with increased frequency even among apparently immunocompetent individuals. At the present time, however, there is no uniform diagnostic and therapeutic approach to improve the unfavorable outcome of patients suffering from sporadic PCML (1,2,3). Even the classification of this neoplasm is still a matter of debate.

Retrospectively, a series of 54 patients with sporadic PCML has been reevaluated. In all cases a low-risk neuroimaging-stereotactic serial biopsy with histological and immunomorphological techniques was performed. The PCML were uniformly classified with the support of immunocytochemical data. In the series presented these tumours have been predominantly classified as high-grade blastic B-cell lymphomas. For that reason this type should be regarded as the prevalent variant of malignant brain lymphomas (1,4). The evaluation of possible prognostic factors suggest that age at admission and morphological features of regression are relevant determinants of survival time. A correlation between neuroradiological tumour size, glucocorticoid administration and morphological signs of regression has been found. The results of treatment in this series suggest that aggressive therapy consisting of irradiation including the whole brain and the meninges at a dose of 50 to 54 Gy or a combination of radiotherapy and chemotherapy improves life expectancy in younger patients (under 60 years), but not in older individuals. The same is true if morphological features exhibited only slight signs of regression.

Because of the lack of uniformity in management of this rare brain neoplasm, different treatment protocols, however, are not comparable, and hence new treatment approaches have not been satisfactorily determined. Therefore, on the basis of our data, a rational diagnostic strategy for PCML is recommended:
First, in patients complaining of a short duration of neurological symptoms consistent with the presence of an intracranial mass, a careful history and thorough physical and neurological examinations are mandatory. Secondly, a neuroradiological examination (CCT or MRI) should be performed. Thirdly, single or multiple circumscribed homogeneous contrast-enhanced lesions requires hospitalization with routine laboratory tests, electrocardiogramm, chest x-ray and CT-stereotactic serial brain biopsy. Prior to CT-stereotactic brain biopsy, corticosteroids should not be administered in order to avoid or reduce tumor regression as well as to facilitate and to ameliorate lymphoma diagnosis and classification, unless herniation is imminent. If the histo- and immunomorphological findings result in the diagnosis of a malignant lymphoma, a routine staging procedure should be performed including chest and abdominal CT-scan, bone marrow aspiration, differential blood count, plasma protein electrophoresis and an assessment of the immune status of affected individuals. Finally, if there is no evidence of extracerebral manifestations of a non-Hodgkin's lymphoma or of a systemic Hodgkin's disease, the extent of PCML onto the spinal cord should be carified by lumbar puncture with cerebrospinal fluid examination.

On the basis of this strategy, PCML should be rapidly diagnosed, the extent of the disease determined and therapy protocols for future prospective randomized long-term follow up studies should be evaluated.

References

1. Braus DF, Schwechheimer K, Müller-Hermelink HK, Schwarzkopf G, Volk B, Mundinger F (1992) Primary cerebral malignant non-Hodgkin's lymphomas: a retrospective clinical study. J Neurol 239: 117-124

2. DeAngelis LM (1991) Primary central nervous system lymphoma: A new clinical challenge. Neurology 41:619-621

3. Hochberg FH, Miller DC (1988) Primary central nervous system lymphoma. J Neurosurg 68: 835-853

4. Schwechheimer K, Schwarzkopf G, Braus DF, Müller-Hermelink HK, Volk B (1989) Primary cerebral malignant non-Hodgkin's lymphomas. Histological and immunopathological findings on stereotactic brain biopsies. Clin Neuropathol 8: 250

106

INVESTIGATION OF NEUROTOXIC SIDE EFFECTS OF CYTOSTATIC MEDICATION

Claus, D., Beck, E.*, Gmeiner, H.J., Puschmann, E., Brunhölzl, C., Jäger, W.*, Neundörfer, B.
Dept. Neurology , * Dept. Gynecology Univ. Erlangen-Nürnberg, Germany

Among different cytostatic drugs Vinblastine, Cytarabine, Procarbazine as well as Cisplatin cause symmetric sensory polyneuropathies. The polyneuropathy caused by Cisplatin starts with distal symmetric paraesthesia followed by overall impairment of sensation. Vibration perception is affected early in the course of the disease. Symptoms develop gradually and in 10% of the cases cranial nerves are also impaired. The clinical picture is not different from that of paraneoplastic polyneuropathies which are seen in up to 33% of cases with ovarial carcinoma (Croft and Wilkinson 1965). The recovery after cessation of the treatment is very slow and often incomplete. Recently results have been published about a preventive effect of the additional medication of an ACTH-analoge (Hovestadt et al. 1992). It was therefore of interest to assess peripheral nerve impairment under Cisplatin treatment by using noninvasive methods.

A group of 70 patients was investigated in a follow up study. 52 patients (59±13yrs.) suffered from ovarial carcinoma (proved by histology), 18 had a mamma carcinoma (48±9yrs.). They all were investigated neurologically. Additionally thermal thresholds and vibration perception were investigated at the ankle by the method of limits (Claus et al. 1990). Patients with ovarial carcinoma received cytostatic treatment with Cisplatin either 50 mg/m^2 (low dose) or 100mg/m^2 (high dose) per course combined with Treosulfane (5g). Patients with mamma carcinoma received different treatment but no Cisplatin and no neurotoxic medication. During four courses patients with ovarial carcinoma reached cumulative Cisplatin doses of up to 300 mg/m^2.

At the first investigation before treatment a distal symmetrical polyneuropathy was diagnosed in 6/52 cases with ovarial cancer (12%). No polyneuropathies were seen in patients with mamma carcinoma. In the follow up study of patients with ovarial cancer 1/4 patients with low and 6/12 with high dose Cisplatin developed a polyneuropathy. There was no significant alteration seen of the blood cell count.

In the investigated group polyneuropathies associated with ovarial cancer were less frequent than in the literature. During treatment a polyneuropathy developed in 1 case with mamma carcinoma. In ovarial carcinoma the manifestation of polyneuropathy was correlated with the Cisplatin dose. Vibration thresholds showed a clear correlation with the cumulative dose of Cisplatin. This was not seen with thermal perception. Vibration perception was impaired before clinical symptoms became manifest. The unimpaired thermal thresholds are in accordance with a neurotoxic affect sparing thinly and unmyelinated nerve fibres. The investigation of vibration thresholds by the method of limits is a sensitive tool for follow up in toxic polyneuropathies.

References:

Claus D, Hilz MJ, Neundörfer B (1990) Thermal discrimination thresholds: a comparison of different methods. Acta Neurol Scand 81: 533-540

Croft PB, Wilkinson M (1965) The incidence of carcinomatous neuromyopathy in patients with various types of carcinoma. Brain 88: 427-434

Hovenstadt A, van der Burg M, Verbiest H, van Putten W, Vecht C (1992) The course of neuropathy after cessation of cisplatin treatment, combined with Org 2766 or placebo. J Neurol 239: 143-146

This work was supported by the Marohn Foundation.

107

Clinical application of [18]FDG-PET for brain tumour grading

R. J. Seitz[1], G. Schlaug[1], A. Kleinschmidt[1], G. Reifenberger[2], W. Wechsler[2], A. Wirrwar[3], B. Nebeling[4].
Departments of [1]Neurology, [2]Neuropathology and [3]Nuclear Medicine, Heinrich-Heine-University Düsseldorf, and [4]Institute of Radiochemistry, Research Center Jülich, FRG.

In neurological patients with brain tumors, the most critical issue is to estimate the tumor biology. Computed radiation tomography (CT) and magnetic resonance imaging (MRI) provide important non-invasive information to identify brain tumors already in-vivo. These methods reveal the tumor location, space occupying character, and disturbances of the blood-tumor barrier. Tumor classification and grading is, however, a domaine of the neuro-pathological examination of tumor tissue. In this study, we examined the usefulness of metabolic measurements using [^{18}F]2-fluoro-2-deoxy-D-glucose ([18]FDG) and positron emission tomography (PET) for grading gliomas in-vivo.

We studied thirty patients with neuropathologically confirmed gliomas of which 6 were glioma recurrences. After intravenous bolus injection of about 5 mCi [18]FDG, tracer uptake in the brain was recorded dynamically for 65 mins using the SCANDITRONIX PC4096 camera [3]. The arterial tracer and glucose concentrations were measured from arterialized venous blood samples (oxygen saturation > 90%). Quantitation of [18]FDG accumulation in tumor and brain tissue was based on the graphical method [2]. Since the abnormal glucose metabolism within brain tumors excludes the use of standard rate constants and since the lumped constant is unknown in human gliomas, no attempts were made to estimate the regional metabolic rate of glucose. Tumor tissue for neuropathological classification was obtained by open surgery (19 patients) or stereotactic biopsy (11 patients).

Our results show that dynamic [18]FDG-PET provided important biological information to characterize brain tumors in-vivo. In general, isomorphic astrocytomas (grade II) had a [18]FDG accumulation rate in the range of cerebral white matter, whereas anaplastic gliomas (grade III) had a high [18]FDG accumulation rate that in some cases even exceeded that of gray matter structures. In glioblastomas, the ring-like tumor borders that were clearly visible in contrast MRI were metabolically active, whereas low [18]FDG uptake occurred in the necrotic center of the tumor. Assuming that the viable tumor rim of glioblastomas had a proliferation rate at least as high as that of anaplastic gliomas (grade III), the relatively low [18]FDG accumulation in the tumor rim was possibly an underestimation due to the limited spatial resolution of the PET scanner. In addition, anaplastic tumor components and high grade tumor recurrences that were not recognized by CT and MRI could be identified by dynamic [18]FDG-PET.

In conclusion, dynamic [18]FDG-PET appears helpful in grading human brain tumors in-vivo in spite of the reported regional heterogeneity of the energy metabolism within brain tumors [1]. In a clinical setting, [18]FDG-PET allows to monitor patients with low-grade gliomas or patients after tumor resection. Furthermore, it appears as a tool for guiding stereotactic biopsy to the most active tumor portion.

References

1. Herholz K, Heindel W, Luyten PR, denHollander JA, Pietrzyk U, Voges J, Kugel H, Friedmann G, Heiss WD (1992) In vivo imaging of glucose consumption and lactate concentration in human gliomas. Ann Neurol 31: 319-327
2. Patlak CS, Blasberg RD, Fenstermacher JD (1983) Graphical evaluation of blood-to-brain transfer constants from multiple-time uptake data. J Cereb Blood Flow Metab 3: 1-7
3. Rota Kops E, Herzog H, Schmid A, Holte S, Feinendegen LE (1990) Performance characteristics of an eight-ring whole body PET scanner. J Comp Ass Tomogr 14: 437-445

108

Neurophysiological Assessment of Pain Pathways in Patients with Brainstem Lesions

R.-D. Treede[1], H.C. Hansen[2] and K. Kunze[2]
1: Institute of Physiology, 2: Neurological Clinic,
University Hospital Eppendorf, D-2000 Hamburg 20, Germany

Laser-evoked potentials are a new clinical neurophysiological tool to study the functional integrity of pain pathways (for review see Bromm and Treede 1991). They have been demonstrated to be useful in the assessment of patients with dissociated sensory loss and have already found wide applications in lesions of peripheral nerves and the spinal cord (Bromm et al. 1991, Kakigi et al. 1992, Treede et al. 1991). We now studied patients with lateralized brainstem lesions, in order to establish the role of laser-evoked potentials and conventional SEPs in the assessment of the functional organization of afferent pathways in the brainstem.

Methods
In each patient, two skin areas were tested: the affected area and a contra-lateral control area. Brief radiant heat pulses (20 ms, 20 W, 20 mm²) generated by a carbondioxide laser were given with randomly interspersed electrical stimuli to the median or tibial nerve. The EEG was recorded from the vertex versus linked earlobes with a bandpass of 0.1-70 Hz. Averages of late evoked potential components were calculated off-line after EOG-artefact rejection (n=40). Median and tibial nerve SEPs were recorded with standard methods.

Results
In two patients with unilateral obliteration of the posterior inferior cerebellar artery (incomplete Wallenberg syndrome) and a corresponding hypalgesia on the contralateral body side, we found a complete loss of laser-evoked potentials from the affected areas. In contrast, conventional median nerve SEPs were normal on both sides, indicating a preferential affection of pain pathways at the brainstem level.

In one patient suffering from brainstem encephalitis, presumably due to herpes simplex virus infection, we were able to demonstrate the success of a high-dose anti-viral therapy. This patient had been severely hypalgesic on the right body side during the peak of the disease. Although at the time of the first recording recovery of pain sensitivity had already begun, laser-evoked potentials were reduced in amplitude by 70% on the affected side. Latencies were normal. The tibial nerve SEPs were normal bilaterally. In a follow-up study 3.5 years later, a complete recovery of sensory function was demonstrated, including recovery of the laser-evoked potentials.

In contrast, one patient with a vascular lesion of the upper brainstem and corresponding vertical gaze impairment was free of sensory loss. In this patient, we found normal laser-evoked potentials and normal SEPs bilaterally.

This sample demonstrates that evoked potentials elicited by painful laser radiant heat pulses can be useful also in patients with brainstem lesions of vascular and inflammatory origin. Laser-evoked potentials provide sensitive parameters for follow-up studies.

References
1. Bromm B, Treede RD (1991) Laser evoked cerebral potentials in the assessment of cutaneous pain sensitivity in normal subjects and in patients. Rév Neurol 147: 625-643

2. Bromm B, Frieling A, Lankers J (1991) Laser-evoked brain potentials in patients with dissociated loss of pain and temperature sensibility. Electroenceph clin Neurophysiol 80: 284-291

3. Kakigi R, Kuroda Y, Takashima H, Endo C, Neshige R, Shibasaki H (1992) Physiological functions of the ascending spinal tracts in HTLV-I-associated myelopathy (HAM). Electroenceph clin Neurophysiol 84: 110-114

4. Treede RD, Lankers J, Frieling A, Zangemeister WH, Kunze K, Bromm B (1991) Cerebral potentials evoked by painful laser stimuli in patients with syringomyelia. Brain 114: 1595-1607

109

DIRECT ACTIVATION OF NICOTINIC ACETYLCHOLINE RECEPTOR CHANNELS BY ANTIBODIES OF PATIENTS WITH MYASTHENIA GRAVIS.

J.Bufler+, K.V.Toyka§, A.Maelicke⁰, Ch.Franke+, +Neurologische Klinik der TU München, Möhlstr.28, 8000 München, §Neurologische Klinik der Universität Würzburg and ⁰Insitiut für Physiologische Chemie und Pathobiochemie der Universität Mainz

Muscle weakness in myasthenia gravis (MG) is caused by a chronic attack of antibodies against the nicotinic acetylcholine receptor (nAChR), resulting in loss of nAChRs of the postsynaptic membrane. It was assumed that the polyclonal antibodies of patients with MG do not directly affect the function of nAChR channels. Using the patch-clamp technique we now have discovered that nAChR channels can be activated by very low concentrations of monoclonal antibodies directed against the acetylcholine binding site and by IgG fractions of patients with MG

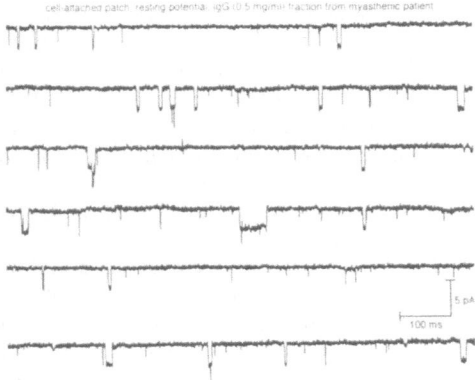

Fig.1 Activation of the nicotinic acetylcholine receptor channel by IgG fraction of patients with MG. The patch clamp technique was applied in the cell-attached mode. If IgG fractions of patients with MG were added to the physiological solution in the patch clamp pipette, current pulses were observed, produced by cations flowing through the pore of an open channel. The dependence on membrane potential of the current amplitude and the mean open time of the channel corresponded to the values obtained with acetylcholine in the patch clamp pipette. We concluded, therefore, that the antibodies activate the nAChR channel. A similar activation was observed with monclonal antibodies against the binding site of the nAChR (WF6) in concentrations above 10^{-13} M

At higher concentrations of antibodies, the nicotinic acetylcholine receptor channels were inactivated in a fashion resembling the desensitization by acetylcholine. These findings, demonstrating a specific, receptor activating and desensitizing effect of an antibody are of fundamental relevance under two aspects: 1. Antibodies stabilize the nAChR in the desensitized state. This antagonistic effect can explain rapid fluctuations of muscle weakness in MG. In addition, the rapid recovery after removal of antibodies by plasmapheresis cannot be caused by newly synthesized nAChRs, but by recovery of desensitized nAChRs after dissociation of antibodies. The complete block of synaptic transmission observed in myasthenic crisis which cannot be influenced by cholinesterase inhibitors may be produced by an inactivation of almost all nAChRs by antibodies. 2. A new molecular mechanism was discovered which may account for rapid changes of electrical properties of neurons in response to the immune system.

110

HETEROGENEOUS AUTOIMMUNE RESPONSE TO ACETYLCHOLINE RECEPTOR IN MYASTHENIA GRAVIS.

A. Melms [1], G. Malcherek [1], H. Link [4], H. Kalbacher [3], J. Lindstrom [5], J. Oksenberg [6], L. Steinman [6], C. Müller [2].

Department of Neurology [1], Medicine [2] and Biochemistry [3], University of Tübingen, Germany; Department of Neurology [4], Karolinska Institute, Stockholm, Sweden; University of Pennsylvania [5], Philadelphia, PA, USA; Stanford University [6], Stanford CA, USA.

The acetylcholine receptor (AChR) of the motor endplate of skeletal muscle is the autoimmune target in myasthenia gravis (MG). AChR is a complex protein antigen containing numerous antigenic epitopes. Immunogenicity of AChR is T cell dependent, hence, autoimmune AChR-specific T cells are required to provide helper signals for autoimmune B cells to secrete autoantibodies to AChR which eventually impair neuromuscular transmission. Experimental evidence from animal models has suggested that autoreactive T cells recognize a limited number of epitopes of an antigen thereby using restricted T cell receptor genes.

We examined the autoimmune T cell response in MG patients and healthy donors after stimulation of peripheral blood lymphocytes with a recombinant AChR α subunit in vitro. AChR α subunit specific T helper cell lines were raised from patients and healthy donors. Although AChR specific T cells were present in the T cell repertoire of healthy donors, the precursor frequency was increased in patients. Using truncated fragments of the α subunit, we found that the majority of T cell lines recognized epitopes on the extracellular part of the molecule. Multiple HLA DR specificities were involved in the recognition of AChR fragments. However, HLA DR3 which is increased among MG patients and contributes to the susceptibility to develop MG was not preferentially used as restriction element. In addition, analysis of the T cell receptor gene usage of AChR-specific T cells was performed by the polymerase chain reaction using specific oligonucleotid primers for variable Vα and Vß gene segments. Acetylcholine receptor-specific T cells from different donors used individual combinations of Vα and Vß gene segments for autoantigen recognition. Some T cells shared antigen specificity or HLA restriction elements, however, there was no association with epitope specificity or HLA restriction element. There was a predominance of certain Vα or Vß families such as Vα8 in MG patients and Vß12 in a healthy donor. In different individuals, Vα8 was associated with different Vß elements. Accordingly, T cells with different Vα8/Vß combinations had different fine specificities as well as different HLA restriction molecules.

Our results extend earlier observations and demonstrate the heterogeneity of the cellular immune response in myasthenia gravis with respect to AChR antigen fragments, HLA restriction molecules and T cell receptor genes in the recognition of the AChR α subunit. These have important implications in designing selective immunotherapies to eliminate autoimmune T cells.

111

Effects of motor training with hemiparetic patients. Threedimensional motion analysis.

T. Platz, P. Denzler, K.-H. Mauritz
Klinik Berlin, Dep. of Neurol. Rehabil. at the Freie Universität Berlin

Introduction: Even hemiparetic patients with almost complete clinical recovery often face unexpected problems when returning to their jobs and families. Knowledge about specific impairment of motor performance and motor learning with these patients is still lacking. Therefore, in this study stroke patients with minor paresis were given a three-dimensional motor learning task.

Method: 20 stroke patients with minimal residual central paresis of their arm were examined (9 pts. with RHD, 11 pts. with LHD; 17 pts. with ischemic stroke, 3 pts. with localized ICB; 10 female, 10 male; age 56.4 yrs., s.d. 10.3 yrs.). A group of 16 non brain damaged control persons was matched for age, sex and intelligence.

Under standardized conditions the seated subjects were asked to make iterative triangular movements of specific configuration and spatial orientation without vision imaging their index finger being a pencil and drawing on a board. Motion was analysed using an optoelectronic system (SELSPOT II; 1 LED; 100 Hz) before and after kinesthetic training with a triangular stencil (20 training movements, 50% guidance). For measuring retention, SELSPOT recording was used again 1 day later. (5 movements each time). The motion analysis system allowed the simultaneous documentation of both configurational and time-dependent parameters.

Nonparametric statistics were used. Immediate and lasting effects were documented for each group by comparing performance before training with performance after training or 1 day later respectively.

Results:

For experimental and control group no right-left differences were found with few exceptions when testing performance after training.

Significant inter-group differences after training were not found for the mean values of the following parameters: velocity, jerk cost, size of triangle, angles and spatial orientation. However, movement time (MT) and acceleration-zero-crossings (AZC) were increased with hemiparetic patients. In addition, for both configurational and time-dependent parameters consistency with movement iteration was reduced: hemiparetic patients showed a higher variability of angles, MT, AZC, and jerk cost.

Experimental and control group showed qualitatively similar learning effects (increase of MT; decrease of mean velocity, variation of mean velocity with movement iteration, and jerk cost; the "drawn" triangles' angles closer resembled the stencil's angles), largely without retention.

Training effects significant only for hemiparetic patients include: increase of break-duration at the triangles' corners; increase of AZC and their variation with movement iteration; decrease of variation of mean velocity.

Analysing training effects using relative changes revealed a higher increase of MT and AZC for hemiparetic patients.

Conclusion: As expected on clinical grounds the examined hemiparetic patients showed similar motor performance and learning as the healthy control group. However, using 3D motion analysis specific (residual) impairment of both motor performance and learning could be demonstrated: hemiparetic patients even with almost complete recovery showed an increased demand for (information processing) time (MT) and possibly for correction of movement directions (AZC) to achieve the behavioral goal. The observed reduction of movement consistency is also in agreement with the hypothesis of a reduced automation of motor control.

112

Patterns of sensorimotor deficits after focal brain lesions

Binkofski F., Kunesch E., Kuhlmann H., Hefter H., Freund H-J., Dept. of Neurology, Heinrich-Heine-University Düsseldorf

It is common clinical experience that residual clinical deficits after stroke correlate only loosely with the site and size of the lesion as shown by MRI scans. The disturbances of hand function after motor stroke are usually attributed to paresis and spasticity with clumsiness and awkwardness of hand movements. Clinical examination shows that in many cases the pattern of deficits comprises other components such as disturbances of coordination (ataxia, dysmetria), of motor plan (apraxia), and use (neglect). Since the significance of these disturbances for the residual motor capacity of the hand can not be assessed properly on clinical grounds, we have designed a test battery for their quantitative evaluation. This comprises examination of: 1. basic motor functions (rapid isometric contractions, tremor, tapping), 2. force control (maximal force, force stability, force tracking), 3. position control during natural hand movements (exploratory movements, pointing, grasping), 4. motor exploration in the right and left hemifield, 5. rhythm production, 6. somatosensory neglect. In addition, Motor and Somatosensory Evoked Potentials were recorded. The results were then correlated with the site and size of the lesion. For this purpose proton weighed MRI slices (scan width 8mm) were analysed by means of a Macintosh computer using "image" program software. Analysis of the lesion was based on standard brain slices of the Talairach Atlas.

The results show, that most motor strokes are complex disorders of motor behaviour consisting of variable proportions of the above mentioned motor dysfunctions. In addition to paresis and spasticity, motor neglect, apraxia and secondary effects of sensory disturbances on motor functions represent the most frequently associated deficits.

The correlation with the lesion site shows that the different motor dysfunctions can be allocated to different areas. It is concluded that different brain modules contribute specific components to intact motor behavior which represents the network activity of various functional subsystems.

References:

1. Freund H-J (1992) The Apraxias. In Asbury, McKhann, McDonald (eds) Diseases of the Nervous System: Clinical Neurobiology (2 ed.) W.B. Sanders Company, Philadelphia; Volume I. pp 751-767.
2. Pause M, Kunesch E, Binkofski F, Freund H-J (1989) Sensorimotor disturbances in patients with lesions of the parietal cortex. Brain 112: 1599-1625.

113

Cortical hypometabolism and striatal necrosis in a patient with temporal lobe epilepsy

A. Weindl, H. Boecker[*], T. Kuwert[*], T. Mayer, B. Winkler, B.U. Meyer, H. Gräfin von Einsiedel, H. Herzog[*], L.E. Feinendegen[*], B. Conrad
Neurologische Klinik der Technischen Universität München und [*]Forschungsanlage Jülich

To evaluate structural-functional relationships in temporal lobe epilepsy the regional metabolic rate of cerebral glucose consumption (rCMRGlc) was measured in a 19 years old patient using ^{18}F-fluorodeoxyglucose PET scanning. This patient had psychomotor seizures which could not be sufficiently controlled with anticonvulsive drugs. Except for a slight rigidity in her left extremities she presented no neurological signs. Cranial CAT and MRI scans showed a nearly complete necrosis of striatum and pallidum of supposed perinatal origin. In the EEG delta- and theta-waves predominated in central, temporal and occipital regions of the right side. Somatosensory and auditory evoked potentials were normal. Visually evoked potentials revealed slightly longer latencies of P_{100} on the right side. Magnetic stimulation over the right premotor and motor cortex revealed a lower threshold, shorter latency and higher amplitude as compared to the left side. Neuropsychological testing demonstrated a deficit in spatial orientation and object recognition. PET scanning demonstrated a lack of signal in the right caudate and thalamus and hypometabolism in the right frontal, parietal, occipital and temporal cortex, whereas CAT and MRI scans did not present side differences in the medial temporal lobe, thalamus and cerebral cortex. Hypometabolism in the medial temporal lobe (hippocampus) is indicative of focal activity in psychomotor epilepsy. Hypometabolism in all cortical areas of the right side which showed no structural abnormalities in CAT and MRI scans may be caused by ipsilateral striatal necrosis.

114

MEASUREMENT OF AUTOMATED HAND MOVEMENTS TO QUANTIFY DOPAMINERGIC EFFECTS IN DE NOVO PATIENTS WITH PARKINSON SYNDROME

G. Arnold, T. Eichhorn, N. Mai, T. Gasser, C. Marquard, W.H. Oertel
Dept. of Neurology, Klinikum Großhadern, University of Munich, 8000 Munich 70

The early diagnosis of Pakinson's disease (PD) is based on clinical symptoms: rest tremor, akinesia and bradykinesia; amelioration of symptoms following therapy with dopaminergic drugs strongly supports the clinical diagnosis. We studied the objective effect of these drugs in early phases of the disease using a computer assisted system.

Patients and methods

We investigated 39 patients with previously untreated Parkinson syndrome ("de novo" patients), six patients with PD and fluctuating response to l-dopa therapy, eight patients with Parkinson syndromes of different etiology (vascular lesions, multiple system atrophy, progressive supranuclear palsy) and 49 control persons. Prior to apomorphine injection, all subjects draw circles of 3 to 5 cm diameter in a fluent counter-clockwise fashion with a high repetition rate for 3 seconds, using a special writing stylus, connected to a digitizing board (TDS ZedPen). Sampling frequency was 166 Hz, accuracy was 0.25 mm in x and y axis.
We repeated analysis 30 min after s.c. injection of 2 - 5 mg apomorphine. We analyzed peak acceleration and acceleration changes per circle using a microcomputer. The result was compared to 30 items of part III of the Unified Parkinson's Disease Rating Scale (UPDRS).

Results

Control persons had acceleration changes between 1.0 and 1.4 per circle. Before injecting apomorphine, all patients had significantly higher values up to 4.0. After the injection of apomorphine those "de novo" patients improved, i.e. had a reduction of acceleration changes, who showed a beneficial effect of oral l-dopa therapy during the follow-up period. This holds also for patients with fluctuating response to l-dopa. On the other side, there was no improvement or even deterioration in those patients who did not respond to oral l-dopa therapy either previously to the apomorphine injection or during a six months follow up period. We observed a high correlation between improvement in automated hand movements and improvement in UPDRS.

Summary

A computer assisted analysis of automated hand movements shows similar sensitivity compared to clinical observation measured by part III of UPDRS even in early stages of the disease; but it is easier to handle and faster to employ.

115

CORTICAL INHIBITORY EFFECTS IN EPILEPSY

K. J. Werhahn, J. Fong, J.C. Rothwell, S. Shorvon, P. D. Thompson and C. D. Marsden.
MRC Human Movement & Balance Unit, Institute of Neurology, Queen Square, London WC1N 3BG, U.K.

Inhibitory mechanisms may play an important role in limiting the spread of cortical potentials in epilepsy. Ferbert et al. (1990) and Kujirai et al. (1991) described new methods of investigating cortical inhibitory mechanisms in intact humans by applying pairs of transcranial magnetic stimuli over the motor cortex.

We now describe experiments using these methods to assess cortical excitability in a 27 year old woman with focal epilepsy since aged 16. She usually has left focal motor seizures followed by secondary generalisation. There are no other seizure types or isolated grand mal. Seizure frequency was 2 per year and at the time of the study she was taking carbamazepine 200mg bd. In the past EEG showed occasional generalised spike waves with no consistent focus of lateralization; CT was normal.

With ethical commitee approval the experiments were conducted using two Novametrix Magstim 200 stimulators. Both stimulators were connected to figure-of-eight shaped coils which were placed over the motor cortex of one hemisphere to test intracortical inhibition or both hemispheres to test interhemispheric inhibition. At intervals from 1 to 16 ms after a conditioning stimulus a second stimulus (test stimulus) was given to the same area to test intracortical inhibition or over the contralateral hemisphere to test interhemispheric inhibition. Surface EMG responses were recorded from the contralateral first dorsal interosseous muscle at rest. Ten trials at each interstimulus interval (ISI) were randomly intermixed with ten test stimuli. Responses were compared by measuring the peak to peak amplitude.

The results showed that at some intervals local intracortical inhibition and interhemispheric inhibition was less than normal. Local intracortical inhibition was decreased at ISI of 2-5 ms for right hemisphere and 3 ms for left hemisphere stimuation. Comparison of the two hemispheres revealed less intracortical inhibition at ISI of 4-5 ms on the right ($p<0.005$, t-test) and at 3 ms on the left suggesting an asymmetry between the two hemispheres. Interhemispheric inhibition of the right (abnormal) hemisphere (from the left) was less than viceversa at ISI of 10-16 ms ($p<0.05$, t-test).

The abnormalities of both tests were more prominent on testing the hemisphere in which seizure began. The fact that there were abnormalities also for the left hemisphere with intracortical inhibition may mirror the frequent generalised epileptic activity in this patient. The results may have been influenced by the patients antepileptic medication, which could enhance cortical inhibition. Assuming that these inhibitory mechanisms either reflect a recurrent inhibition from pyramidal cell collaterals or cortico-cortical inhibitory processes (Kujirai et al. 1991) we suggest that there are changes of intracortical inhibitory mechanisms in patients with epilepsy of focal onset. The technique may be useful in the study of cortical excitability in epilepsy.

References

1. Ferbert A, Priori A, Rothwell JC, Colebatch J, Day BL, Marsden CD (1990) Trans-callosal effects on motor cortical excitability in man. J Physiol 429: 38P
2. Kujirai T, Sato M, Rothwell JC, Day BL, Thompson PD, Wroe S, Asselmann PT, Marsden CD (1991) Inhibitory interactions between transcranial brain stimuli applied over the motor cortex in man. Society of Neurocience 17: 1023P

116

Psychogenic seizures: diagnosis by suggestive provocation

J. Bauer, C. E. Elger, G. Hefner, and V. Güldenberg

Klinik für Epileptologie, Universität Bonn
Sigmund Freud Str. 25, D-5300 Bonn, Germany

The differentiation between epileptic and psychogenic seizures is of high clinical importance. In many cases the description of the seizure obtained from the patient or witnesses does not permit its classification. Interictal EEG findings have only limited diagnostic value since many patients with epilepsy develop psychogenic seizures in the course of their disease. These can either occur in addition to persisting organic seizures or after ceasing of the latter. In 1982 Cohen and Suter [1] recommended a suggestive provocation for diagnosis of psychogenic attacks. We performed provocations in 80 patients with suspected psychogenic seizures (49 women and 31 men, aged between 25 and 66). Prior to the procedure patients were informed about the possibility to provoke a seizure by injection of a "convulsivum" and about its possible blocking by an "antidot". Simultaneous video- and telemtric EEG recording permitted to register the reactions of patients after they had been administered 5-10 ml of the "convulsivum" i.v. (NaCL + Cytobion). In 63 patients a psychogenic seizure was provoked in this manner and was then interrupted by an "antidot" (NaCl). In 5 out of those 63 patients provocation was only successful after the second attempt. Typical features of psychogenic attacks are closed eyes, abrupt (tonic) falling, arhythmic cloni (preferably of the lower limbs), paraesthesia of the limbs and ceasing of symptoms after application of an "antidot". EEG recordings during the attacks never showed epileptiform activity. The recorded seizures were demonstrated to the patients and their families, in order to get them identified as the patients' "typical" seizures. In 75 % of these cases we thus succeeded to identify psychogenic seizures by means of suggestive provocation. In some of these cases the diagnosis had previously remained unclear for years or even decades.

Reference

1. Cohen RJ, Suter C (1982) Hysterical seizures: suggestion as a provocative EEG test. Ann Neurol 11: 391-395

117

Prolactin in Focal Epilepsy

H.Meierkord (1), S.Shorvon (2), St.Lightman (3) and M. Trimble (2).

(1) Humboldt-Universität Berlin, Medizinische Fakultät (Charité), Neurologische Klinik, Schumannstraße 20/21, O-1040 Berlin
(2) University Department of Clinical Neurology, National Hospital for Neurology and Neurosurgery, Queen Square, London WC1N 3BG
(3) Neuroendocrinology Unit, Charing Cross and Westminster Medical School, London

The acute effects of partial (focal) epileptic seizures on serum prolactin levels were studied in two groups of patients: (1) 10 with temporal lobe seizures and (2) 11 with seizures that arose from the frontal lobes, recorded on cable video-electroencephalographic telemetry. Six of the eight complex partial seizures of temporal lobe origin were associated with a marked rise in prolactin levels at 10 minutes after onset (rise in levels, from a mean of 279 to 534 mU/L), compared with a rise in only one of the eight frontal lobe complex partial seizures. None of the five simple partial seizures (two of temporal and three of frontal lobe origin) was associated with a marked rise in prolactin levels. This difference in prolactin response following complex partial seizures of frontal and temporal lobe origin may help in the clinical differentiation of these seizures. A failure of prolactin levels to rise does not, however, exclude a diagnosis of complex partial seizures; thus, this measurement will not help in the clinical differentiation of frontal lobe complex partial seizures from psychogenic attacks.

118

Clinical Value of Proximal Conduction Block Studies

Jaspert, A.; Claus, D.; Spitzer, A.; Grehl, H.; Neundörfer, B.
Department of Neurology, University of Erlangen

Proximal nerve segments cannot be stimulated reliably by conventional stimulation techniques. Transcutaneous supramaximal stimulation of motor roots and proximal parts of motor nerves, however, can be performed by a high-voltage, low output impedance stimulator (Digitimer D 180) with a stimulus of short rise time. As the distance between proximal stimulating points cannot be measured exactly, no reliable values for proximal conduction velocities can be obtained. Electrophysiological evidence of conduction block or abnormal temporal dispersion, however, may reveal conduction abnormalities also in proximal localization. In acquired inflammatory demyelinating neuropathies, demyelination is usually multifocal in contrast to the more generalized demyelination in hereditary neuropathies. To increase the probability of recording focal demyelination, proximal conduction block studies were applied to 17 patients with inflammatory neuropathies of different origin. Twelve patients presented with typical acute or chronic inflammatory demyelinating polyradiculoneuropathy (AIDP, CIDP), 3 patients with atypical chronic neuropathies, 1 with vasculitis of the peripheral nervous system and 1 with radiculitis. Surface recordings from the abductor digiti minimi and tibialis anterior muscles were performed after stimulation of the ulnar nerve at wrist, distal and proximal of the elbow, axilla, Erb`s and C7, and of the peroneal nerve at fibula head, sciatic notch and L1.

Conduction block or abnormal focal temporal dispersion could be observed in one or more nerve segments in all patients. Thirteen patients revealed conduction block or temporal dispersion in proximal localization. The patients with atypical neuropathy did not show any signs of demyelination in electrophysiological routine tests. In these patients, proximal conduction block or proximal temporal dispersion were the only pathological electrophysiological findings. Conduction blocks in other locations than the typical entrapment sites were also found in the patient with vasculitis of the peripheral nervous system and were probably caused by ischemic lesions. Direct compression of the nerve must also be considered in the differential diagnosis of conduction block. Proximal conduction block studies were repeated in 4 patients with chronic inflammatory demyelinating polyneuropathy after high-dose intravenous immunoglobulin therapy. As early as 2 days after the beginning of therapy conduction block disappeared, corresponding to an increase in muscle strength.

In conclusion, proximal conduction block studies are a useful tool in detecting focal demyelination. They should be performed especially in patients supposed to have inflammatory neuropathies with normal results in routine examinations of distal nerve segments. By proximal conduction block studies, the evidence of possibly treatable neuropathies might be increased.

119

STANDARDIZATION OF SIMPLE AND COMPLEX SOMESTHESIS.

Henningsen, H. (1), Pause, M. (2), Depts. of Neurology, University of Heidelberg (Klinikum Mannheim) (1) and Würzburg (2)

Neurological rehabilitation is widely defined as a specific therapy for a neurological deficit. While this approach has been used for many years successfully for example in the treatment of aphasia, there are only very poor descriptions of specific therapeutic strategies for patients with disturbance of somesthesis. This might be due to the lack of a congruent classification and standardization of somesthetic performance, especially of complex somesthetic deficits and their consequences for motor ability. While standard values of a normal population for touch, pressure or thermal and pain sensitivity exist, there are no descriptions of the respective values for semi-complex (e.g. roughness discrimination, dynamic two-point-discrimination, directional sensitivity), somesthesis or complex somatosensory performance (stereognosis, spatial size discrimination, tactile reading like Braille). It was the aim of the study to design a test set applicable for standardization of somesthesis in normals and in patients with hypesthesia.

In the literature as well as in own pilot investigations threshold approximation methods were shown to be poorly reproducible in the critical range, therefore it is necessary to us the method based on the signal detection theory described by Johnson (1980). With this strategy a statistically acceptable discrimination index for each quality can be determined. A disadvantage, however, is the long duration for the many comparisons of paired stimuli. Cognitive factors as "Gestalterkennen" do not or only to a minor degree have an influence on the discriminative performance.

After having tested a normal population of 80 subjects of different age groups we would recommend to use light touch (tested with Semmes-Weinstein monofilaments) as a representative quality for simple somesthesis . For evaluation of semicomplex somesthesis the test of roughness discrimination of exactly defined nylon-print patterns is practicable. Complex performance can be tested by size discrimination of pairs of simple objects or relief figures with identical proportions. To exclude generalized attentive disturbances, a d2 test must be done with every evaluation.

The testing of the 80 normal subjects resulted in nonsignificant sex differences and only few significant age-dependent differences in simple and complex somesthetic qualities. These and the correlation of the performances of simple/semicomplex/complex sensibility (and additional motor) tests are evaluated for possible clinical use.

Literature:

Johnson KO (1980) Sensory discrimination: Decision process. J Neurophysiology 43: 1771-1792

120

Computer-stereotactic treatment of tremor types resistant to therapy

F. Mundinger, J. Schwab
St. Josefskrankenhaus, Freiburg i Br, Germany

Drug treatment of therapy-resistant advanced parkinsonism-related tremor, essential (hereditary) intention tremor, and action myoclonus (cerebellar) tremor (e.g occurring in multiple sclerosis and postinjury) is unsatisfactory, partly due to the unwanted side effects it can cause. Graft techniques, which are still in the experimental stages, have shown no effect on the tremor associated with Parkinson's disease. Therefore, in such cases thalamo-subthalamotomy is still the treatment of choice. The method involves coagulating the disinhibited cerebellar afferent pathways (rubro-dentato-thalamic) and the impulses from Mollaret's triangle (dentato-rubro-inferiore olive and back). They run via the radiatio prelemniscalis in the subthalamic zona incerta to the thalamic ventralis oralis posterior nucleus (V.o.p) and to the nucleus intermedius (V. im.) (Haßler, Riechert, Mundinger 1956). Here we coagulate the afferent pathways to the motoneurons of the premotor and sensomotor cortices, whose effector in the cortico-spinal tract conducts impulses to the periphery. Electrode positioning is guided with our original stereotactic universal system (Mundinger and Riechert 1956) using modern computer-guided imaging techniques (Mundinger and Birg 1961). Coagulation is done in the anatomically adapted structures in the zona incerta (Mundinger 1963) and at the base of the posterior oral ventral nucleus and nucleus intermedius. Lesioning of the nuclei and pathways is done using a computerized temperature-controlled high-frequency lesion maker (Neuromed 50*). The use of different types of electrodes (string-stick electrodes with a variety of insulated tips and diameters), depending on the intraoperative effect, while the patient is awake reduces the lesion volume and shape in comparison with the earlier methods of pallidotomy and lesioning of the oral nucleus, thus minimizing risks. From a total of 4,400 patients operated on for tremor in the last 40 years, 1,680 patients operated on between 1975 and 1985 were evaluated. Mortality was 0.25%, the rate of persisting complications was 1.01%. Out of 1,243 operations (2,144 extremities) in patients with parkinsonism-related tremor, depending on the lesioning depth (e.g. the subthalamotomy and basal V.o.p and V. im.) complete tremor relief was achieved in 62% (directly postsurgery 92%) and improvement in another 19%. After V.o. thalamotomy and pallidotomy, 65% experienced tremor relief and 17% marked reduction, with progression in only 6 to 9%. Essential (hereditary) intention tremor after a mean follow up of 8.7 years (range 1 to 20 years) was relieved or reduced in 72% of 105 patients, an up to 50% improvement was achieved in another 9.4%. Tremor remained unchanged in 14% and worsened in 4.7%. Intention tremor showed no change on the non-operated side in 54.3% and increased in 26%, yielding a total of 80.3%. A long-term evaluation (3 to 10 years) showed that action myoclonus tremor in a total of 84 cases was relieved or considerably reduced in 51%, moderately or slightly reduced in another 33%. This is an impressive outcome, since in only 14 (2%) was no improvement or worsening observed in the long-term evaluation. The results show that computerized stereotactic temperature-controlled high-frequency coagulation in the thalamus and subthalamus is still the treatment of choice for treatment-resistant tremor of various etiologies.

*Leibinger and F.L. Fischer, 7800 Freiburg i. Br.

Authors: Professor Fritz Mundinger, M.D.
former Director of the Department of Stereotaxy and Neuronuclearmedicine, University of Freiburg, and Jan A. Schwab, M.D.
St. Josefskrankenhaus, Freiburg i. Br., Germany

121

Effects of High-dose Intravenous Immunoglobulins in Patients with Chronic Guillain-Barré-Syndrom

Grehl H, Jaspert A, Claus D, Neundörfer B.
Dept. of Neurology, University Hospital, D-8500 Erlangen, (Germany)

Chronic Guillain-Barré-Syndrom (GBS) is characterized by a chronic progressive or relapsing and remitting course of demyelinating polyradiculoneuropathy. Neurophysiological tests such as conduction block studies as well as antiglycolipid antibodies, examination of cerebrospinal fluid and nerve biopsy can be helpful to distinguish these cases from inherited or degenerative neuropathies or to separate different subgroups. Recently various groups have been described including typical chronic inflammatory demyelinating polyneuropathy (CIDP) according to the criteria of the "Ad Hoc Subcommittee of the AAN AIDS Task Force" [1], multifocal motor neuropathy, lower motor neuron syndromes and motor CIDP [2]. Atypical demyelinating neuropathies, however can also be observed.

An immunologic basis has been suggested in all cases of chronic GBS; beneficial effects of corticoid therapy, plasma exchange, chemotherapeutic drugs or a combination treatment regimen were observed in most of these patients. However, this therapy may cause serious side effects, particularly when long-term administration is necessary. Another group of patients, on the other hand, is refractory to therapy. Recent evidence suggests that intravenous administration of high-dose human immunoglobulins may be helpful in some cases of chronic GBS and few side effects are known so far.

We report on 11 Patients including 8 with chronic progressive and 3 with relapsing demyelinating polyneuropathy. Six patients revealed a typical CIDP, one a multifocal motor neuropathy and 3 an atypical neuropathy with focal demyelination. Other therapeutic regimen given before had shown no or only moderate effect in two patients; some patients exhibited serious side effects of this therapy. After 400 mg immunoglobulin per kg body weight per day given intravenously for 5 days no effect could be observed in 2 patients. In 9 patients the symptoms ameliorated within two weeks, in 7 of these within the first 3 days. One of these patients did not respond to other immunosuppressive drugs before. In all patients symptoms reoccurred after 1-9 weeks. Following 3 - 18 months of therapy, 9 patients now have no or only very slight symptoms. They receive one day immunoglobulin every 1-6 weeks. During 88 months of therapy no serious side effects occurred. No correlation was found between duration or course of the disease and effects of therapy.

High-dose intravenous immunoglobulin therapy is an effective therapeutic regimen in chronic GBS. Although in some patients there are no beneficial effects, some cases improved, in whom previous therapy with prednisone had failed. Even though only few side effects are known, careful follow-up examinations are necessary during long-term treatment.

References:
1. Ad hoc subcommittee of the AAN AIDS Task force (1991) Research criteria for diagnosis of chronic inflammatory demyelinating polyneuropathy (CIDP). Neurology 41: 617-618

2. Pestronk, A (1991) Motor neuropathies, motor neuron disorders, and antiglycolipid antibodies. Muscle Nerve 14: 927-936

122

Clinical course of a polyradiculitis over 900 days

Günther T, Kaendler SH, Enzensberger W, Fischer P-A
Department of Neurology, University Hospital Frankfurt/M, Germany

We report on a case of Guillain-Barré syndrome in a 60 year old patient. On October 11, 1989, spending his vacations in Reno (Nevada, USA), the patient developed a polyradiculitis during an acute respiratory infection on top of underlying asthma. The disease took a rapidly progressive course and the patient had respiratory failure on the second day. He was intubated and required assisted ventilation. Within the first 2 weeks 8 plasmapheresis treatments were given, without therapeutic effect on the severe muscle weakness.

On November 11, 1989, the patient who was still on respiratory support was transferred by airplane to the Neurological Intensive Care Unit (ICU) of Frankfurt/M University Hospital. Tracheotomy was performed. Diagnosis of Guillain-Barré syndrome was confirmed by repeated lumbar puncture. After one year the patient showed first signs of motor recovery. Up to now pareses have not completely resolved, but the patient is able to lift his arms to a 45 degrees angle and to sit in a special wheel chair. He has generalised muscle atrophy. Since he received intensive physiotherapy, only slight joint contractures have developed.

The patient suffered multiple complications in the course of the disease. These included numerous pneumonias, accompanied by pleural empyema and fistula, leg vein thrombosis, pulmonary emboli, myocardial infarction, chronic constipation as a symptom of autonomous nervous system involvement, and allergic skin reactions.

On March 3, 1992, the patient was transferred to a neurological rehabilitation center. Because of recurrent pneumonia he had to be readmitted to our ICU. After his respiratory situation was stabilised discharge to his home was prepared, which took place on July 13, 1992. The patient still requires a ventilatory support for several hours daily because of pulmonary fibrosis. The patient's medical insurance therefore provided a home respirator. The patient is being cared for by his wife and also receives outpatient nursing care.

The clinical course, especially the various complications and the stepwise preparations of discharging the patient home are discussed. The psychological development of the patient and his wife from initial apathy and depression to a more active attitude and finally demand for discharge is presented.

123

NEUROCYSTICERCOSIS: CSF AND SEROLOGICAL DATA IN THE-RAPY CONTROLLING

G. Holzer, M. Raitzig, J. Müller, A. Haaß, K. Schimrigk
Universitätsklinik, Klinische Neurochemie, 6650 Homburg

Introduction: Infections with taenia are curiosities nowadays since the meat inspection was legally directed. The cause of infection can be uncontrolled production of meat or lies in tourism wide over the world. Man as host of taenia saginata or taenia solium can tolerate the relatively weak symptoms. The cys ticercosis as stage of worm fins in contrast is a real threatening disease. Many organs may be affected. The infection of brain induces an autochthonous immunologic defense reaction. Recently we diagnosed a neurocysticercosis in one of our patients and surveyed the effect of the therapy on CSF parameters and immunity of the patient with serological methods.

Patient and methods: A 48 years old patient had been admitted in a foreign hospital with symptoms headache and somnolence which were mainly caused by an acute hydrocephalus. After an extern drainage in order to release the intracranial pressure the patients condition improved. He was then adopted in our clinic for further diagnostic attempts. The suspected parasitic infection of the CNS was confirmed by serological study of the blood serum and the CSF. Findings of the Bernhard Nocht Institute in Hamburg indicated cysticercosis. The subsequent therapy with Praziquantel (50 mg/kg/day) started in the 5th week after the first symptoms. In the first CSF which was got in the 4th week, before therapy, we found an inflammatory cell reaction with 260/3 cells/ul and an autochthonous IgG synthesis proved by IgG index and isoelectric focussing on PAG. CSF parameters and the specific antibody reaction were controlled in the 3 months after the beginning. We determined the titers of antibodies against cysticercus and echinococcus in CSF and blood serum with a home made ELISA with sandwich technique and horse radish peroxydase as marker enzyme. The antigens were friendly gifts of the B. Nocht Institute in Hamburg, dir. Prof. Dr. Mannweiler.

Results and discussion: Both cell count and protein concentration showed a rising trend, persisting after therapy. In the 7th week lymphocytosis with the maximal cell count in the course of the study was seen (740/3/ul). After 3 months the cells in the CSF had decreased (128/3/ul). A loss of autochthonous IgG was indicated by the IgG index falling from 2.2 in the 4th week to 1.0 in the 7th week. In the 13th week the IgG index had slightly risen again to 1.1. The IgM index fell continuously from 0.5 to a value of 0.2 (normally lower than 0.08). The differences of CSF oligoclonal IgG banding in the course of our study were not marked. The trend of the specific antibody index (IAI) was in correlation with the IgG index. The serum titer against cysticercus fell continuously after therapy meanwhile the IAI as measure of the intrathecal antibody quantity passed a minimum in the 7th week and climbed up again (36, 22, 26). This could mean that a consumption of antibodies was induced by a therapeutical antigen release. High serum titers against the echinococcus antigen showed a remarkable cross reaction of serum antibodies with the two antigens. With echinococcus crossreacting parts of the antibodies in the CSF were clearly smaller than in serum, the IAI were in the range between 2 and 4 compared with cysticercus IAI in the range of 22 to 36. In relation to serum a varying antigen specificity of autochthonous antibodies is argued.

124

Psychiatric and psychosocial problems in patients with intractable complex partial seizures prior to and following epilepsy surgery

G. Hefner[1], C. E. Elger[1], J. Zinner[1], and S. Kasper[2]

[1]Klinik für Epileptologie and [2]Klinik für Psychiatrie
Universität Bonn, Sigmund Freud-Str. 25
D-5300 Bonn, Germany

Epilepsy surgery improves the possibility to treat patients suffering from intractable complex partial seizures. In a high percentage complete relief from seizures can be obtained. This, however, can cause new psychiatric and psychosocial problems. The aim of our study is therefore to systematically investigate the influence of temporal lobe epilepsy surgery on the psychiatric and psychosocial situation of the patients. To that purpose we developed a standardized psychometric procedure consisting in physician-rated and self-report inventories and semi-structured questionnaires prior to surgery and at 6 and 12 months postoperatively. 30 patients were investigated, 16 women and 14 men, aged between 15 and 55 years. 13 had a left temporal, 17 a right temporal lobectomy. 10 out of 30 had an intracerebral lesion (1 cavernoma, 1 angioma, 1 subarachnoidal cyst, 4 astrocytoma, 2 oligodendroglioma, 1 mixed glioma). The results did not show a uniform picture. Preoperatively thought disturbances such as slowness of thoughts were predominant. Postoperatively there were marked effects on levels of depression and activation in those 21 patients who were free of seizures. Those 9 patients who did not become seizure free after surgery did not show any significant changes as compared to their presurgical situation. The main problem reported by the patients postoperatively was the complete reorientating in the psychosocial field resulting from the new situation. Adaption to a seizure free life is demanded from the patients as well as from their surrounding. In summary we therefore favour a psychotherapeutic guidance of the patients and related persons prior and following epilepsy surgery. Further investigations with an increased number of patients [1] are neccessary to confirm these results.

Reference

1. Naugle RI, Rodgers DA, Stagno SJ, Lalli J (1991, Unilateral temporal lobe epilepsy: an examination of psychopathology and psychosocial behavior. J Epilepsy, 4:157-164)

125

The Use of Sedatives and Analgesics in brain
injured Patients in controlling the Levels of
Plasmacatecholamines

H.J.Stuerenburg, M.Hase, P.Hinse, P.Neunzig,
K.Kunze

University Hospital, Hamburg-Eppendorf
Neurological Department

Patients with severe brain injuries frequently
exhibit an increase of plasmacatecholamines and
metabolites as a result of the deregulation of
autonomous centers. One set of consequences leads
to considerable cardiovascular deregulation, while
centrally released noradrenaline gives rise to
tertiary brain damage by means of various
mechanisms. In particular, through cellular
swelling, there is a rise in intracranial pressure
and, therefore, an increase in ischaemia.

Methods : 8 patients between the ages of 24 and 78
yrs. old were examined with severe brain injuries.
Initial Glascow-Coma Scale : 3 - 8.
A generalized brain edema was exhibited by 5
patients.
7 patients were provided with an epidural pressure
transducer. Plasma samples were taken daily by
arterial catheters and were analysed through
High-Pressure Liquid-Chromatography with
electro-chemical detection.
Levels of noradrenaline, adrenaline, MHPG and HVA
were determined.

Results : A significant negative correlation was
demonstrated in all patients between the level of
plasmacatecholamines and the use of analgesics and
sedatives (Fentanyl, Midazolam). The average
maximum value of noradrenaline was 791 +- 162
mg/dl. The suppression of higher levels of
noradrenaline to a normal level (240 mg/dl in
resting patients) was achieved through different
applications of sedative / analgesic perfusion
(calculated from the linear regression curve drawn
from the relationship between noradrenaline
concentration and sedative / analgesic dosages).
The necessary sedative/analgesic dosage for
individual patients was between 0.02 mg/h Fentanyl
+ 1,32 mg/h Midazolam and 0.51 mg/h Fentanyl +
31,96 mg/h Midazolam. The average value was 0.18
mg/h Fentanyl + 11,41 mg/h Midazolam (+- 0.07 mg/h
Fentanyl + 4,34 mg/h Midazolam).

In conclusion, the most important factor effecting
the level of plasmacatecholamine in brain injured
patients is the applied dosage of the sedative /
analgesic perfusion. It is not, as was demonstrated
here, the neurological data which is based on the
topographical situation of the contusions or the
measured intracranial pressure.

126

ANALYSIS OF THE HEART RATE VARIABILITY AND ATROPINE-INDUCED HEART RATE ALTERATIONS IN PATIENTS WITH BRAIN STEM LESIONS

Weis, M., Claus, D., Rechlin, T., Hilz, M.J.
Neurological Department, University Erlangen-Nürnberg, Germany

Introduction:
The cardiac autonomic innervation is very complex. The central control is maintained by the brain stem, hypothalamus and other suprabulbar centers, which regulate cardiac output and its situative adjustment over the vagal and sympathetic nerves. The periodic heart rate variability is mainly controlled by the parasympathetic nervous system. Therefore, brain stem lesions, for example lesions in the vagal nuclei region, are able to cause autonomic dysregulation. As patients with autonomic dysfunction are known to have a high risk of cardiovascular complications, they require intensive cardiac monitoring.

Material and Methods:
25 patients (15 men, 10 women) aged 19 to 78 years (mean age 54 years) in the neurological ICU suffering from ischemic brain stem lesions were investigated by analyses of the periodic heart rate variability. First, the variability of heart rate was evaluated at rest. ECG was recorded, digitalized and stored on a personal computer. Data were evaluated using programs, which automatically detect the QRS complex and measure the R-R intervals. Mean heart rate (HR), variation of the R-R intervals, variation coefficient (VC) and RMSSD (root mean square of successive differences) are calculated out of 150 artefactfree intervals. The reaction of HR to atropine was tested in 88% of the cases using intravenously administered doses of 0.5 or 1.8 mg (0.6 mg/ml/min) atropine sulfate. ECG was monitored during injection and the following 15 minutes and the maximal change in HR from rest was calculated.

Results:
The mean HR at rest was 93.0 BpM, the mean variation of RR intervals was 12.5 BpM. The VC was pathologically diminished in 64% of the patients, the RMSSD in 60% and both, VC and RMSSD, in 52%. The HR of the patients with diminished VC and RMSSD was significantly higher (104.4 BpM) than that of the patients with normal results (74.7 BpM) ($p < 0.001$; Wilcoxon). The mean change of HR was 14.3 BpM following injection of 0.5 mg atropine sulfate (8 patients) and 26.9 BpM after doses of 1.8 mg atropine (14 patients). 80% of the patients with pathological results at rest had diminished heart rate responses to atropine. In all patients with normal VC and RMSSD HR increased more than 35 BpM.

Conclusions:
Autonomic dysregulation with impaired control of the heart rate could be demonstrated in patients with brain stem lesions. Comparing results at rest and atropine induced reactions, there are corresponding pathological or normal results in most of the cases. If there are borderline results at rest, the "atropine test" may have discriminating functions.

Platform session III
Prevention in neurology

127

Paradoxical embolism via the patent foramen ovale – A probable cause for cryptogenic stroke in the young

Christopher Doherty, Andreas Stockmanns, Jan-Hinnerk Weingärtner, Frank Peter Job*, Peter Hanrath*, Erich Bernd Ringelstein

Departments of Neurology and Cardiology* Klinikum RWTH, University Hospital, Pauwelsstr., D-5100 Aachen, Germany

Seven to 55% of ischemic strokes amoung young adults remain etiologically unclaryfied. Lechat and co-workers (N Engl J Med 1988; 318:1148-52) recently had focussed attention on paradoxical embolism via the patent foramen ovale as a more important cause for stroke in the young than previously thought.

In order to clarify whether patent foramen ovale (PFO) with subsequent paradoxical embolism of microbubbles into the middle cerebral artery (MCA) is significantly more frequent in young stroke patients than in age-matched normal controls, a series of 77 patients with ischemic stroke below the age of 45 years (including 3 TIAs) were reinvestigated in 1991 by means of transesophageal contrast echocardiography (TEE) and, simultaneously, by transcranial Doppler sonography (TCD) of the MCA. Eight to 10 ml of an agitated saline solution were injected into the right antecubital vein. Patients had consecutively been collected from 1985 to 1987 and had been classified etiologically as either "clarified" or "unclarified" according to the initial clinical and laboratory findings. For further analysis, two patients with congenital ventricular septum defects and one patient with congenital atrial septum defect were excluded. A group of 46 healthy young adults aged 21 to 51 years served as normal controls. During TEE, only 11 patients out of the "clarified" group (11/33; 33%) had PFO, but significantly more so out of the "non clarified" group (23/41; 56%, p = 0.029). In general, PFO was seen in 44% (34/74) of all young stroke patients, and in 43% (20/46) of normal controls. The rate of positive findings increased by 20% under Valsalva manoeuvre in that 30 patients presented canalisation of microbubbles into the MCAs under these conditions. The passage time from the end of the intravenous injection till the occurrence of bubbles into the MCA lasted from 4 to 9 seconds. During TCD of the MCA, paradoxical cerebral embolism again occurred significantly more frequently in etiologically unclarified stroke patients (22/41; 54%) than in the claryfied group (8/33; 24%; p = .017). There was a good correlation of positive findings during TEE and subsequent embolism of microbubbles into the MCA (phi = .713, maximum possible value .924).
We conclude that PFO is significantly more frequent in young stroke patients with unidentified stroke etiology than in those with obvious causes of stroke (e. g. atherothrombosis and dissections of the carotid arteries, or embolic heart disease). In the general stroke population, however, PFO does not seem to be more frequent than in healthy controls. Findings strongly suggest an etiological role of PFO in the cryptogenic type of stroke in the young due to paradoxical embolism.

128

IS ASPIRIN DANGEROUS IN CAROTID ARTERY STENOSES ?

Widder B, Kleiser B, Dürr A
Neurologische Universitätsklinik Ulm, W-7900 Ulm, FRG

During the last years, Aspirin has found widespread use in the treatment of atherosclerotic cerebrovascular disease. Its acceptance is based on numerous publications dealing with the value of antiplatelet treatment in the prevention of stroke. On the other hand, however, several reports doubt about its effectiveness in the presence of internal carotid artery (ICA) stenoses.

1. RETROSPECTIVE RESULTS

Methods: In 171 carotid thrombendarterectomies the surgical specimens were investigated macro- and microscopically (8). The intraplaque morphology was subdivided into predominantly fibro-atheromatous tissue, friable atheromatous debris and intramural hemorrhage. An intramural hemorrhage was only assumed, if the hemorrhage made up at least 50 % of the plaque thickness. In addition, the clinical documentations were analyzed or the family doctors were asked whether the patients took Aspirin during the last months before surgery.

Results: 38 out of the 171 cases showed relevant intramural hemorrhage. 48 revealed friable atheromatous debris, which may be interpreted as relic of a remote intramural hemorrhage. A tendency towards an association between the presence of complex plaques (debris, hemorrhage) and Aspirin treatment could be found (Fig.1). The correlation, however, was not significant (p>0.05).

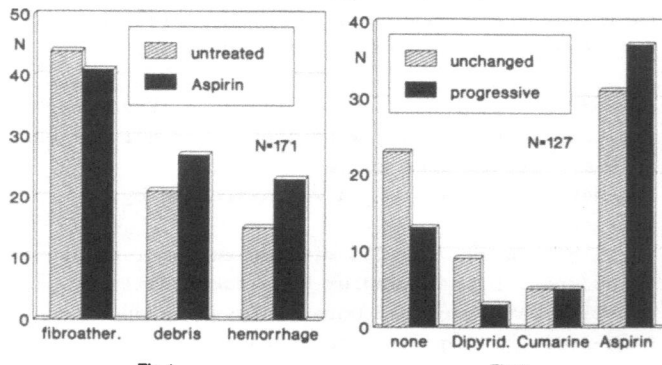

Fig.1   Fig.2

2. PROSPECTIVE RESULTS

Methods: 127 patients with 161 ICA stenoses with initial diameter reductions between 40 and 80 % were followed in 6 month intervals clinically and sonographically. At each reinvestigation the patients were asked for the actual use of drugs, especially antiplatelet treatment.

Results: During the follow-up of 46 months 44 stenoses showed relevant progression of more than 10 % diameter reduction. In addition, 19 patients developed middle or high grade stenoses on the initially non-stenosed side. Patients treated with Aspirin or Cumarine showed a higher progression rate as compared to those without antiplateted treatment or dipyridamole administration (Fig.2). The correlation, however, is only roughly significant (p=0.05). Six of seven patients, who developed an occlusion of the initially stenosed carotid artery, took Aspirin at the time of the occlusion. Of these, one developed a minor stroke, one a TIA.

DISCUSSION

Similarly to other studies in the literature, we are not able to give a conclusive answer to the question, whether Aspirin treatment in ICA stenoses is beneficial or not. While ERNST et al. (4) did not find any correlation between antiplatet therapy and plaque morphology, ABURAHMA et al. (1) reported a significant association between Aspirin and multiple intramural hemorrhages. The subgroup analysis of the AITIA trial (5,6) did not reveal a higher stroke rate in medically treated patients. On the other hand, CARSON et al. suggested that Aspirin was responsible for the progression to severe stenosis in most of their patients. Moreover, CHYATTE and CHEN (3) reported a high incidence of stroke in Aspirin treated patients without warning TIA.

In conclusion, the aim of our paper is drawing attention on the still unresolved questions concerning Aspirin treatment in higher grade ICA stenoses. Until studies with larger series are available (7), uncritical antiplatelet administration in such patients should be avoided. In particular, since progression of carotid artery stenoses compromises an increased risk of stroke, patients with relevant ICA stenoses treated with Aspirin should be closely followed by Doppler ultrasound at least in 6 month intervals.

REFERENCES

(1) Aburahma AF et al. (1989) Am Surg 55 : 169-173
(2) Carson SW et al. (1981) Surgery 90 : 1084-1092
(3) Chyatte D and Chen TL (1990) Neurosurgery 26 : 565-569
(4) Ernst RL et al. (1986) Stroke 17 : 540-541
(5) Grotta JC et al. (1984) Neurology 34 : 437-442
(6) Lemak AL et al. (1986) Neurology 36 : 705-710
(7) The Asymptomatic Cervical Bruit Study Group (1991) 48 : 683-686
(8) Widder B et al. (1990) Ultrasound Med Biol 16 : 349-354

129

Anticardiolipin Antibodies in Oculocerebral Ischaemia and Migraine: Prevalence and Prognostic Value.

Paul Hinse; Antje Schulz; Friedrich Haag; Manuel Carvajal; Andreas Thie. Neurologische Universitätsklinik Hamburg.

Introduction: The presence of antiphospholipid antibodies (APA) has been associated with a variety of neurological disorders including focal cerebral ischaemia, retinal ischaemia and migraine. The prevalence of APA in patients with cerebrovascular disease varies considerably between reports, and data concerning the prevalence of APA in migraine patients are limited. The prognostic importance of APA in patients with oculocerebral ischaemia (OCI) is unknown. We prospectively studied the prevalence and prognosic value of anticardiolipin antibodies (ACLA) in patients with acute or chronic OCI and in patients with migraine.

Methods: Seventy-two consecutive patients with acute or chronic OCI (29 women, 43 men; mean age: 51.2 yrs., range: 18–81 yrs.) and 25 patients with migraine (22 women, 3 men; mean age: 30.3 yrs., range: 18–52 yrs.) were enrolled. In 53 patients with acute OCI, ACLA assays were performed within the first 4 weeks after the index event. In 19 patients with a history of brain ischaemia timing of ACLA-assays varied from 4 weeks to 2 years after the index event which was defined as the most recent cerebrovascular incident with complete neurological evaluation. Quantitative determination of ACLA was performed by ELISA.

Results: Thirty-two of 72 patients with OCI (44%) showed weakly positive ACLA titers (IgG/IgM < 20 GPL/MPL–U/ml), highly positive ACLA titers (IgG/IgM > 20 GPL/MPL–U/ml) were found in 9 patients (12,5%). ACLA were detected in 53% of 36 young patients under 50 years of age and in 61% of 36 older patients. History and CT scan findings gave evidence of recurrent cerebral ischaemia in 6 of 31 ACLA–negative patients (19%), in 7 of 32 weakly positive patients (22%) and in 6 of 9 patients with highly elevated ACLA titers (67%). Fifteen of 25 patients with migraine (60%) had weakly positive (12) or highly positive (3) ACLA titers.

Discussion: In our assay we considered a test positive if an ACLA level above 2 standard deviations of a mean reference value was detected, i.e., beyond the 95% percentile of the log–normal distribution in 1483 healthy blood donors. We found a remarkably high prevalence of ACLA in our patients: 57% of the patients with OCI and 60% of the migraineurs showed elevated ACLA titers. However, only in 12,5% of the patients with OCI, ACLA titers were above 20 GPL/MPL–U/ml. In this group of patients recurrence of brain ischaemia was significantly more frequent than in patients with negative or weakly positive ACLA titers (p = 0.0133).

ACLA can be detected in young, aswell as in older stroke patients. In our series ACLA prevalence rates did not differ significantly in patients above or below 50 years of age.

Our results suggest that highly positive ACLA titer in patients with OCI are associated with increased risk for recurrent brain ischaemia whereas detection of weakly elevated ACLA in patients with OCI probably is of no prognostic importance.

Whether ACLA play a role in pathogenesis of migraine or are a marker for stroke risk in migraineurs remains to be determined.

130

Aspirin responder and Aspirin non responder - a two year follow up

K.-H. Grotemeyer*, H.W. Scharafiniski** , I.W. Husstedt* - Department of Neurology, University of *Münster & **Essen, F.R.G.

Introduction:

Aspirin (ASA) is proposed to be effective in stroke-prophylaxis because platelet prostanoid-pathway is completely inhibited by ASA. Platelet reactivity (PR) is normalized by ASA as well. However 12 hours later about one third of stroke patients shows a pathological PR again (1). This laboratory phenomena of the secondary ASA non responders may be clinically relevant.

Methods:

138 of the 180 patients included initially in the study, (53 female 85 male) age 58 ± 15 years, suffering from stroke of the internal carotid artery territorial treated with acetylsalicylic acid (aspirin) (3 x 500 mg) were observed over a period of 24 months. Before discharge from hospital platelet reactivity was determined 12 hours after oral administration of 500 mg aspirin in each patient.

Results:

36 of the 180 patients included in the study discontinued medication because of gastric side effects. 83 of the 138 patients showed a normalized platelet-reactivity under aspirin treatment. Pathologically high test values were found in 55 patients (aspirin non responders). 18.1% of the 138 analyzed patients showed one of the study principal parameters; 10 patients suffered a second vascular event before the end of month 24 and another 15 patients died in consequence of a second vascular event during the observation period. During the two year observation period one of the study principal parameters was seen in 3.4% of the aspirin responders and in 40% of the aspirin non-responders (chi-square = p<0.00001).

Conclusions:

The simple division of aspirin treated stroke patients into aspirin responder and aspirin non-responder could be useful in future aspirin studies, because such a classification may lead to a more homogeneous group of observed patients and perhaps to a more conclusive statement on aspirin in secondary stroke prophylaxis.

Reference:

Grotemeyer K.-H. (1991) Effects of acetylsalicylic acid in stroke patients. Evidence of nonresponders in a subpopulation of treated patients. Thrombosis Research 63:587-593

131

Isokinetic strength training in neuromuscular disease

U. Mielke, A. Marian, K. Lederer, C. Mayer,

K. Schimrigk

Universitätsnervenklinik-Neurologie

D-6650 Homburg/Saar

An isokinetic strength training program was applied to the leg muscles of patients suffering from limbgirdle muscular dystrophy (7) and spinal muscular atrophy (4). The training was performed 3 times per week for a period of 8 weeks. Exercise intensity was controlled by repeated maximal strength tests carried out at motion velocities of 60 deg/sec and 180 deg/sec to analyse correlations of coordination and strength according to the Hill coefficient. Exercise effects were evaluated by spiroergometry with special regard to ventilation and oxygen consumption. Before and after each training unit serum values for CK and myoglobin were determined. The average increase in muscle strength in the muscular dystrophy group was 34% both at low and high motion velocity. 12 weeks after termination of the training program the strength gain was still 25% compared to the baseline values. In the muscular atrophy group, however, the increase in strength was different with respect to the motion velocity. Using 60 deg/sec a strength gain of 45% was obtained while at 180 deg/sec the increase was only 22%. This difference is highly significant (p < 0,01). A feasable explanation could be that similar to muscular dystrophy in motor neuron disease the remaining fibers keep their trainibility as far as strength is concerned but are much more impaired with respect to intermuscular coordination due to reduction in the number of motor neurons. The results suggest that in muscular dystrophy strength and intermuscular coordination may well be improved by isokinetic training methods. In spinal muscular atrophy strength may be trained with similar efficiency while the improvent of intermuscular coordination is limited.

132

Bicycle ergometer tests in diagnosis and therapy of neuromuscular disorders

C. Hartard, S. Scharein, K. Kunze
Neurologische Universitätsklinik, Hamburg,FRG

Introduction
Incremental bicycle ergometer work leads to increasing serum lactate levels due to the additional use of glykolysis in skeletal muscular energy production. The concept of the aerobic-anaerobic threshold (1) was developed from endurance measurements in athletes. Workloads associated with serum lactate levels below 4 mmol/l lead to a lactate-steady-state and can be performed over 30-60 minutes while higher workloads lead to a further serum lactate increase and exhaustion. Therefore the skeletal muscular endurance capacity can be estimated from the mode of serum lactate increase under increasing ergometer workloads in healthy persons. Those workloads associated with serum lactate levels of 3.5 - 4.0 mmol/l are supposed to be the upper threshold for an endurance training. We examined whether bicycle ergometer tests with lactate measurements can also be used in patients with neuromuscular disorders for assessment of their skeletal muscular endurance capacity. In addition we investigated which differential diagnostic information can be gained from lactate levels under incremental ergometer work.

Methods
Patients were first examined in a bicycle ergometer test with increasing workloads of 30 watts every 4 minutes, starting at 30 watts. Heart rates and ear lobe capillary lactate levels were measured every four minutes. In the two following bicycle ergometer tests, patients cycled with constant workloads corresponding to the loads at the 3.5 - 4.0 mmol/l and at the 2.0 - 3.3 mmol/l serum lactate levels in test one over 20 minutes each.

Results
In all three patients with Mc Ardle syndrome, the lactate level remained low but the heart rate increased under rising bicycle ergometer work. In constant bicycle ergometer tests, these patients had no increase of serum lactate levels but an initially increasing and after a few minutes decreasing heart rate corresponding to the "second wind" phenomenon. Three patients with functional muscular symptoms, in whom a muscular disease could be excluded by further examinations, interrupted the increasing workload bicycle ergometer test at lactate levels below 4 mmol/l. But in these patients serum lactate levels and heart rate increased in parallel. In four patients with mitochondrial myopathies, the lactate levels were already elevated in resting state and increased steeply under rising work loads. In 6 of 29 patients with different myopathies and in 9 of 24 patients with different neuropathies, a workload corresponding to lactate levels of 3.5 - 4.0 mmol/l in the rising workload test was adequate for endurance work while in the remaining 23 patients with myopathies and 13 patients with neuropathies the work load adequate for endurance work was lower and corresponded to serum lactate levels of 2.0 - 3.3 mmol/l in the increasing load bicycle test.

Conclusion
Bicycle ergometer tests with measurements of ear lobe capillary lactate levels under increasing and constant workloads can be used in patients with neuromuscular disorders as a screening method for metabolic myopathies. Patients with McArdle syndrome had missing or very low lactate but normal heart rate increases. Patients with mitochondrial myopathies showed elevated lactate values at rest and steep lactate increases under ergometer work of low intensity. Patients with functional muscular symptoms serum lactate levels and heart rates increased in parallel but they interrupted the test at low grade work levels. As in healthy persons the test could be used in patients with neuromuscular disorders for quantitative assessment of skeletal muscular endurance capacity and as a result in physiotherapeutic training and therapy control.

Literature
1. Heck H, Mader A, Hess G, Müller R, Hollmann W (1985) Justification of the 4 mmol/l lactate threshold. Int J Sports Med 6: 117-130

133

KNOWLEDGE ON PHYSIOLOGICAL PERFORMANCE IN SPORTS MEDICINE - BASIS FOR AN IMPROVED DIAGNOSIS AND TREATMENT CONTROL FOR NEUROMUSCULAR DISEASES

H. Rühl[1], U. Mielke[2], A. Wagner[1], K. Schimirigk[2]

1) Clinic of Neurology of the University of Leipzig
2) Clinic of Neurology of the University of Homburg/Saar

The analysis of the motor functions has so far played only a secondary role in the diagnosis and treatment control of neuromuscular diseases. In contrast, years of research in this area have been done in the field of performance diagnosis in sports medicine. In examinations, with the aid of dynamographic and surface electromyographic methods, it was attempted to find relevant parameters to quantify the motor performance capacity. The following parameters proved to be particulary significant for the motor condition (1):

1. The economising quotient. This is determined from the average activity of the agonist and the force produced (unit μV/N) and serves to evaluate the motor efficiency (economy).
2. The endurance quotient. This expresses the percentage changes (deteriorations during performance) in the economising quotient and serves as a measure to assess the motor fatigue.
3. The coordination quotient. This is determined from the average surface EMG activities of agonists and antagonists and provides quantitative details on the occurence of muscular dysbalances.

This was carried out using a polygraphic measuring system, which allows dynamographic (force, speed) and surface electromyographic signals (4 to 6 muscles) under conditions specific to certain sports (telemetry, e.g. canoe racing) to be determined.

Since there was no basis for comparison for the initial stages of the examination, norms for the individual stages of endurance had first to be established. By means of progressive examinations during certain training cycles, the significance of individual parameters was examined and the actual measurements were later used to regulate training. It emerged as a result of these examinations that specific norms have to be worked out for each structure of movement.

These findings now form the basis in neurology for examinations which will enable the diagnosis and assessment of the course of neuromuscular disorders to be improved. An isokinetic measuring and performance system (Biodex Multijoint System) and an equipment to determine the surface EMG signals (Myosystem 2000, Noraxon) are available for these examinations. The current task is to establish dynamometric and electromyographic norms for selected joints with defined conditions for measuring EMG signals and of performance.

Initial examinations on healthy subjects (n=20, students) served this purpose. The data was compared with that of some patients (monoradiculopathies with neurogenic paresis).

Initial findings underline the importance of the motor functional diagnosis to quantify the extent of neurogenic disturbance as a basis and point of reference in assessing the course of neuromuscular diseases and carrying out scientifically sound therapy.

1) Rühl, H., Wittekopf, G. (1984) Possibilities to influence adaptive processes in the motor system in order to characterise sports performance. Medicine and Sport 24: 101 - 104

134

Neurochemical parameters in senile dementia of Alzheimer's type

M. Strittmatter[1], G. Hamann[1], C. Reuner[2] and H. Cramer[2]

[1] Department of Neurology, University of Saarland, D-6650 Homburg
[2] Department of Neurology, University of Freiburg, D-7800 Freiburg

Introduction: In senile dementia of Alzheimer's type (SDAT) changes in several transmitter systems have been described. A deficiency of somatostatin attributable to intrinsic cortical neuron damage seems to be one of the prominent neurochemical features at the beginning of SDAT. Moreover alterations of the molecular forms of somatostatin are noted.

Patients and methods: In 53 patients with SDAT (50 f, 3 m; 85.6 ± 5.8 years) and in an age-matched control group (n=12; 11 f, 1 m; 82.3 ± 6.7 years) somatostatin-like immunoreactivity (SLI), , its molecular forms somatostatin-14 (SST-14), somatostatin-28 (SST-28), high-molecular weight form (HMV-SST) and Des-Ala-somatostatin (Des-Ala-SST) were determined in the cerebrospinal fluid (CSF). SLI was determined using a specific antibody (K-18) raised in rabbits which recognices the somatostatin molecule at the ring structure. SLI was fractionated by reversed phased HPLC using a C18 column. Moreover homovanillic acid (HVA) and hydroxyindoleacetic acid (HIAA) were determined by electrochemical detection. Cognitive impairment was evaluated in all patients by use of the global deteriroration scale of Reisberg (GDS).

Results: Total SLI was significantly decreased to 18.6 ± 8.7 fmol/ml in SDAT compared to control group. The decrease of SLI in SDAT was correlated with dementia scores (r= 0.41, p< 001). After classification according to the stage of deterioration, patients with GDS 5 showed no significant descrease of SLI, while significant decrease was observed in GDS 6 (p<0.05) and GDS 7 (p<0.01). HPLC separation of SLI revealed molecular heterogeneity of SLI. Four peaks were eluted (HMV-SST, SST-14, SST-28 and Des-Ala-SST). In SDAT SST-14 was significantly decreased to $21.4 \pm 13.5\%$ vs. $31.2 \pm 13.6\%$ (p<0.05) whereas HMV-SST was significantly increased to $15.6 \pm 7.1\%$ vs $10.1 \pm 4.9\%$ in controls.

HVA and HIAA were significantly lower only in advanced dementia (GDS). Longitudinal studies in 4 patients (over 2 years) showed similiar results. We observed positive significant correlations between HVA and HIAA in controls (r=0.68) and SDAT (r=0.59). Moreover HVA and HIAA were correlated with SLI (r= 0.59, r= 0.54).

Discussion: In SDAT SLI was significantly reduced in CSF in accordance with numerous earlier reports. Our finding of qualitative and quantitative changes in the molecular forms is compatible with dysregulated synthesis and/or processing of somatostatin in SDAT. It remains to be established whether these changes are specific for the neuropathological processes involved in plaque and tangle formation or reflect a generaliced alteration of protein biosynthesis and posttranslational processing in SDAT. The late and rather moderate decrease of HVA and HIAA in SDAT suggests that the progressive loss of HVA and HIAA in the CSF may be secondary and less specific compared with the change in SLI. In summary neurochemical investigations of the CSF in SDAT could establish an additional and earlier securing of the clinical diagnosis SDAT and give a possibility to control the clinical course.

135

GENETIC COUNSELLING IN AUTOSOMAL-DOMINANT CEREBELLAR ATAXIAS

T. Klockgether, U. Wüllner, D. Petersen, J. Dichgans

Neurologische Klinik und Abteilung für Neuroradiologie, Universität Tübingen, Hoppe-Seyler-Str. 3 , W-7400 Tübingen

The autosomal-dominant cerebellar ataxias (ADCA) comprise the entire spectrum of dominantly inherited, progressive ataxias irrespective of the underlying neuropathology. Harding (1982) proposed to subdivide ADCA into four clinical categories [2]. The most common type (ADCA-I, n = 43) is clinically characterized by the occurrence of additional non-cerebellar symptoms, such as ophthalmoparesis (40 %), pyramidal tract dysfunction (25 %), muscle wasting (17 %), dementia (12 %), bladder dysfunction (10 %) and akinesia (7 %). In contrast, ADCA-III (n = 12) is a pure cerebellar disorder. ADCA-II and ADCA-IV are rare disorders characterized by pigmentary retinal degeneration or myoclonus, respectively.

ADCA usually starts in middle age: mean disease onset was 43.6 ± 12.7 years in ADCA-I and 41.4 ± 11.6 in ADCA-III. Although ADCA is sometimes characterized as a 'late-onset' disorder, an early disease onset does not exclude the diagnosis: in 11% of our patients ataxia started before the age 25 years. Life expectancy is restricted to 18.4 years after disease onset in ADCA-I and 23.5 years in ADCA-III.

The mutation causing ADCA-I has been assigned to chromosome 6 near the HLA-locus (SCA 1 locus) in several families in North America [3,5]. However, linkage to this locus was excluded in families coming from a large population of patients with ADCA-I in Cuba [1] suggesting that ADCA-I is a genetically heterogeneous disorder. Genetic heterogeneity will make it difficult to develop molecular tests for routine presymptomatic diagnostic use. Therefore, genetic counselling must remain restricted to informing affected patients about the 50% risk to transmit the disorder to their offspring. Although patients with ADCA have characteristic findings in elelctrophysiological tests and in magnetic resonance imaging [4], the value of these investigations for presymptomatic diagnosis is unknown.

References

1. Auburger G, Orozco Diaz G, Capote RF, Sanchez SG, Perez MP, Del Cueto ME, Meneses MG, Farrall M, Williamson R, Chamberlain S, Baute LH (1990) Autosomal dominant ataxia: genetic evidence for locus heterogeneity from a cuban founder-effect population. Am. J. Hum. Genet. 46: 1163 - 1177

2. Harding AE (1982) Clinical features and classification of the late onset autosomal dominant ataxias. Brain 105: 1 - 28

3. Rich SS, Wilkie P, Schut L, Vance G, Orr HT (1987) Spinocerebellar ataxia: Localization of an autosomal dominant locus between two markers on human chromosome 6. Am. J. Hum. Genet. 41: 524 - 531

4. Wüllner U, Klockgether T, Petersen D, Naegele T, Dichgans J (1992) Magnetic resonance imaging (MRI) in hereditary and idiopathic ataxia. Neurology (in press)

5. Zhogbi HY, Pollack MS, Lyons LA, Ferrell RE, Daiger SP, Beaudet AL (1988) Spinocerebellar ataxia: variable age of onset and linkage to human leukocyte antigen in a large kindred. Ann. Neurol. 23: 580 - 584

136

Neurological results after chronic exposure to perchlorethylene
- a preventive challenge -

G.Walter, A.Haaß
Neurological department of the University Clinic Homburg/Saar

The risk of damage to the nervous system after occupational exposure to solvents is generally estimated as being low. We examined 12 male workers between the age of 35 and 59 years(average age 47.9 years), who were exposed in a factory disposing of dead animals bodies over a period of 2 to 28 years(average: 11.5 years of exposure) to perchlorethylene. This solvent was applied to chemically remove the fat from the dead animals bodies. The workers were exposed to this solvent up to 12 hours per day by leakages of the pipeline system or when opening the installations for extraction and distillation, or on the occasion of the daily cleaning and repair of blocked pipes. They were also exposed when transporting the bonemeal still containing the solvent and by breathing the air contaminated by the solvent. The workers did not wear any safety clothes. All workers were neurologically and psychologically examined including a nuclear magnetic resonance examination(NMR).

The neurological and psycho-pathological findings showed unobtrusive results in 2 cases. In 5 cases we observed slight pseudo-neurasthenic interferences with unspecific losses of affective reaction and with subjective complaints on concentration and memory losses, on symptoms of fatigue and occasional autonomic-vasomotoric disturbances. In 2 cases we saw more serious losses of intellectual and mnestic-cognitive performance. In 3 further cases we found distinct characteristics of an organic change of personality consisting of affective restriction, of the inability of maintaining control over affective reaction, of psycho-motoric slowness, of coping with new and unexpected situations and perseveration and finally of a lack in drive.

The seriousness of the psychopathological disturbances correlated with the time of exposure: 2 patients with an average of 5.5 years of solvent exposure did not show any psychopathological findings, 5 patients with an average of 10 years of exposure showed pseudo-neurasthenic symtoms and 5 patients with an average of 15.6 years of exposure showed serious losses of mnestic-cognitive abilities and/or organic changes of their personality. The first psychopathological interferences appeared after 3 years of exposure. After 9 years of exposure both regular findings and serious psychopathological interferences could be observed.

In two cases NMR examinations corresponded to the age of the examined persons, in two further cases the NMR examinations resulted in isolated focal changes, in five cases we found cerebral-atrophical changes alongside with focal changes and in three cases we found isolated cerebral atrophies.

Atrophical changes correlated with the seriousness of the psychopathological disturbances and with the duration of the exposure: 4 patients without any atrophy in the NMR were exposed on the average 6.25 (2-11) years, 5 with atrophical changes alongside with focal changes were exposed an the average 11.8 (4-15) years and 3 patients with isolated and serious cerebral atrophies were exposed on the average 18.3 (7-28) years. The earliest point of time to diagnose a cerebral atrophy was after 4 years of exposure, but always after more than 11 years of exposure.

As for their being exposed to solvents, the examinated persons with focal changes did not show any differences to the remaining group: 7 patients with focal changes were exposed on average 14.1 years, 5 patients without focal changes were exposed on average 13.6 years. In 5 out of 7 cases focal changes appeared with simultaneous cardio-vascular diseases or with the additional consume of alcohol, psychopharmaca and nicotine.

Our examinations show an obvious correlation between occupational exposure to perchlorethylene and the appearance of organic cerebral disorders. In face of missing therapeutic possibilities this fact underlines the necessity of taking preventive measures.

Poster session III
Prevention in neurology

137

On the differential diagnosis and classification of blepharospasm

A.O. Ceballos-Baumann, B. Conrad

Neurologische Klinik, Technische Universität München

Blepharospasm (BS) denominates a syndrome characterised by spasms of the m. orbicularis oculi. Here, we refer to a form of focal dystonia in the area of the eyelid closing muscles. Common atypical forms, the waxing and waning character of focal dystonias, modifying sensoric "tricks" and local changes (blepharochalasis, levator-desinsertion), rare and common differential diagnosis (e.g. ocular myasthenia, chronic tic disorders, mono-/achromatopsia) as well as associations with autoimmunune diseases (e.g. ocular myasthenia, dysthyroid ophtalmopathy) often confound ophtalmologists and neurologists. Diagnosis seems to be straightforward, if during the clinical examination chronic intermittent, involuntary forceful eyelid closure is documented. We postulated that a definition of BS as "chronic involuntary, intermittent forceful eyelid closure" is misleading and does not cover the whole spectrum of the disorder. We were also interested in a classification of BS, which may improve the nosology of this focal dystonia.

We analysed the data gained from a standardized questionaire of 127 patients who were initially diagnosed as BS as focal dystonia (96 females, 31 males, mean age 65 females, 62 males, mean symptom duration, 7,0 years females, 6,2 years males). Videotapes could be reviewed in 104 of these patients.

Intermittent, forceful lid closure was documented in 89 patients (70,1%) which in many cases could not be seen on the videotape. 17 patients displayed tonic narrowing of the palpebral fissure and 17 patients had a strong levator-inhibition component as the predominant feature (it has been also called apraxia of lid opening). In one patient with severe psychosis and on long term neuroleptic medication, the course of the disease suggested a stereotypy as the correct diagnosis instead of tardive BS.

The concept of "blepharospasm" remains misleading. It is nosologically more precise to use the term dystonic lid opening disorder or lid closing dystonia. According to our data we suggest the following classification of this focal dystonia: 1. classical blepharospasm- , 2. tonic- and 3. levator-inhibition-type. This classification takes into consideration the wide spectrum of the disorder. It may aid in the differential diagnosis and be useful in establishing more specific guidelines for the therapy of lid closing dystonia.

138

NEW POSSIBILITIES FOR THE NEUROMUSCULAR FUNCTIONAL DIAGNOSIS ON THE ASSESSMENT OF THE COURSE OF NEUROMUSCULAR DISEASES AND CONTROL OF THEIR TREATMENT

A. Wagner[1], H. Rühl[1], U. Mielke[2], H.-J. Zett[1], K. Schimrigk[2]

1) Clinic of Neurology of the University of Leipzig
2) Clinic of Neurology of the University of Homburg/Saar

There are only few findings available for comparison on the question of effectiveness testing of physiotherapy necessary for a projected longer-term study concerned with elaboration quantitative criteria by which the individual functional condition of the neuromuscular system can be determined and described both in a complex way and with subtle differentiation.

Dynamographic and electromyographic methods form the basis of the initial stages of the examination. With the aid of an isokinetic and polyelectromyographic measuring system and under standardized conditions of measurement, recording techniques and muscle performance facts about the force, intermuscular coordination and efficiency of the use of force can be obtained. Conventional and automatic methods of analysis by EMG give information on the activity of motor units. A Biodex-System to record the dynamographic parameter, Myosystem 2000 for the surface electromyography, a needle electromyography system (DANTEC, Counterpoint) and an analogue recorder (DTR 1800) are available.

The examination is currently carried out in three stages. First the force curves are determined under isometric conditions applied to the joint and the surface electromyogram is simultaneously recorded polygraphically from various agonistic and antagonistic innervated muscles. Thus information on the maximum force, speed, endurance and motor efficiency (economy) is gained. In a second examination, these results are completed by simultaneously recording needle electromyogram. Finally, the needle EMG-examinations are carried out from selected muscles and the recruitment pattern and the parameters of motor unit action potentials are separately estimated.
The initial examinations were carried out on the knee joint. The EMG-recordings performed from M. rectus femoris lateralis, M. vastus medialis, M. vastus lateralis and M. biceps femoris. The selection of parameters was standardized for healthy persons (n=20) and compared with the results of patients (n=10) with monoradiculopathy and selected neuromuscular diseases (spinal muscular atrophies, progressive muscular dystrophies).

The aim of the examinations is to quantify the deficit of the neuromuscular functional disturbance, to therapeutically improve the remaining functional capacity and to bring a positive influence to bear on the regenerating processes.

Herpes simplex encephalitis during pregnancy: A 4 year follow-up investigation

Manfred Max Hummel* and Gert Huffmann
Neurologische Universitätsklinik, Rudolf-Bultmann-Strasse 8,
W-3550 Marburg, FRG

An early start in therapy with Acyclovir in herpes simplex encephalitis (HSE) leads to a less marked neuropsychiatric residual condition. HSE in pregnancy is rarely reported. There are in particular hardly any long-term observations of the course of the disease in mother and child.

We report on a pregnant patient in whom HSE had been confirmed by specific IgM-antibody-titres (ELISA) in cerebrospinal fluid. Therapy with Acyclovir was started on the day of admission. The pregnancy was terminated by caesarian section the next day. After 3 3/4 years the patient and her child were examined again. Electroencephalography (EEG) and cranial computerized tomography (CCT) were repeated. In addition serologic investigations were performed on the child.

The 32-year-old patient fell ill in the 35th week of gestation with fever and headaches. Within a few days she suffered from disorientation followed by clouding of consciousness and focal cerebral symptoms consisting of an aphasia and grands maux.
The EEG showed left fronto-temporal periodic delta-complexes. Initially, at this point there were no pathological findings in the CCT, even with contrast medium. The tentative diagnosis of HSE led to the introduction of Acyclovir therapy.

Nevertheless the clinical state of the mother worsened. The next day tachycardia of the fetus made a caesarian section necessary. The maturity of the male newborn corresponded to time of gestation. Apgar score was 8-9-10. Four days later the EEG showed no more periodic complexes, but CCT showed large hypodense areas in the left temporal lobe and two smaller hypodensities on both sides paramedian superior to the corpus callosum. While the temporal finding was typical of focal encephalitis, the two small foci were uncommon for this diagnosis. At the border of the hypodensities an enhancement of contrast medium was seen. Distinction from disorders of the blood-brain-barrier, as seen in ischemic cerebral infarction, was formally impossible (1). So vascular lesions had to be considered in a differential diagnosis.

Six weeks after improvement the patient was discharged with a slight aphasia. She exhibited 3 3/4 years later an elevated emotional state, slight disorders of concentration and memory, and a very slight amnestic aphasia. No further neurological deficits were seen. In the EEG basal activity was normal, and only paroxysmal focal slowings occurred. The CCT showed marked defects in left temporal lobe and insula. Alterations in other areas as well as the dilatation of the ventricles demonstrated that the disease exceeded a focal encephalitis (1).

The son showed no other neurological symptoms than a slight strabism. Serologic investigations on herpes simplex antibodies (ELISA) were negative, thus excluding herpes-simplex-infection of the child. Toxic effects of the medication were seen neither at birth nor during the follow-up investigation of the child.

Rapid disappearance of the delta-complexes in EEG is probably a favourable sign for the prognosis indicating the success of the treatment.

(1) **Hummel MM, Lütcke A, Mertins L** (1991) Klinische, elektroencephalographische und computertomographische Verlaufsuntersuchungen bei der Herpes simplex Encephalitis. In: Huffmann G, Braune HJ (eds.) Infektionskrankheiten des Nervensystems. Einhorn-Presse Verlag, Reinbeck pp 272-276

*Present address and address for offprint requests: Oberarzt Dr. med. M.M. Hummel, Psychiatrische Universitätsklinik, Rudolf-Bultmann-Strasse 8, W-3550 Marburg, Federal Republic of Germany

Impairment of Unilateral Motor Learning by Left Sided Frontomedial Lesion in Man

AW Kornhuber[1], M Becker[1], W Lang[2], M Lang[1], F Uhl[2]
[1]University of Ulm, Dept. of Neurology, Neurophysiol. Section, Oberer Eselsberg, D-W-7900 Ulm, Germany, [2]University of Vienna, Dept. of Neurology, Allgemeines Krankenhaus, Währinger Gürtel, A-1090 Wien, Austria

Introduction: The important role of the frontal lobe for motor learning in higher mammals and man is well established. In previous studies where EEG and SPECT were applied [1,2], we could demonstrate the involvement of both hemispheres of the frontal lobe in learning a horizontal mirror tracking movement. By the means of a morphometric study we now try to further elucidate the question of a critical lesion site for this function.

Methods: From a sample of 55 patients with chronic frontal lobe lesions well documented by computerized tomography those 54 with all necessary data available were selected for analysis. Patients with brain tumors, subarachnoid hemorrhage from aneurysms and other diffuse lesions wore not included in this study. Subjects (Ss) tracked a random polygon path on a computer screen with a small tracking symbol (cross) guided by a manipulandum ('joy stick') with the hand prefered. For the horizontal mirror tracking task the horizontal coupling between manipulandum and symbol was inverted, i.e. the cross moved towards the left when the Ss moved to the right. Eight individual trials of 80 seconds each were performed. The mean distance between target path and tracking symbol (arbitrary units) served as a performance measure. For a global learning index (LI) an average was taken from the first three trials (A), and from the last three trials (B). LI was defined as $LI = (B - A)/A$, i.e. Ss learned, when LI was less than zero. Motor learning was considered to be impaired for $LI > 0$. Lesions were digitized on standard planes taken from [3] (9 successive canthomeatal planes, volume element [VOXEL]: $3mm \times 3mm$ raster, 10mm slice thickness). For each VOXEL the association between lesion and poor test performance was evaluated for the hypothesis of an impairment by a lesion (exact one-sided Fisher test [$p<0.05$]). In order to assess the statistics of the area defined by this criterion with a 'Monte-Carlo' simulation, a random assignment of the label: "impaired motor learning" for different patients of the same number was made 10000 times. For each of these random sets of patients the same procedure as above was applied. Both the number of points found in the area previously labeled, and the sum of $log(p)$ in this area were computed.

Result: Fourteen of the 54 patients had impaired motor learning ($LI > 0$). For a 'significant' ($p < 0.05$) association between impaired unilateral motor learning and a lesion a small volume (23.6 cm³) was found on the left side of the superior frontal gyrus. The 'Monte-Carlo' simulation did not show another random set of patients with a similar result for this volume. For 74.2% no associations were found within this volume, for 98.8% the overlap was less than 10%. Similar results were obtained for the sum of $log(p)$. A significant correlation was found between lesion size in the frontomedial region and LI ($p < 0.05$).

Conclusion: In contrast to the involvement of a larger portion of the human forebrain of both hemiheres in motor learning [1, 2] lesions within a small region in the depth of the left superior frontal gyrus may critically impair motor learning.

Literature:
1. Lang W, Lang M, Kornhuber A, Kornhuber HH (1986) Electrophysiological evidence for right frontal lobe dominance in spatial visuomotor learning. Archives Italiennes de Biologie 124: 1-13
2. Lang W, Lang M, Podreka I, Steiner M, Uhl F, Suess E, Müller C, Deecke L (1988) DC-potential shifts and regional cerebral blood flow reveal frontal cortex involvement in human visuomotor learning. Experimental Brain Research 71: 579-587
3. Matsui TA, Hirano A (1978) An Atlas of the Human Brain for Computerized Tomography. Fischer, Stuttgart

141

High manganese intake from rural well-water is not a risk factor for Parkinsonism

G. Korf (1), P. Vieregge (1), B. Heinzow (2), H.-M. Teichert (3), P. Schleifenbaum (4), H.-U. Mösinger (4)
(1) Klinik für Neurologie und (3) Institut für Medizinische Statistik und Dokumentation, Medizinische Universität zu Lübeck, D-2400 Lübeck; (2) Untersuchungsstelle für Umwelttoxikologie, D-2300 Kiel; (4) Kreisgesundheitsamt Herzogtum-Lauenburg, D-2418 Ratzeburg, Federal Republic of Germany.

Childhood living in rural areas with well-water supply is epidemiologically supposed to be a risk factor for later development of idiopathic Parkinson´s disease; chronic exposure to Manganese (MN) is one of the most common causes of secondary Parkinsonism. A case-control study, therefore, investigated, whether chronic exposure to well-water rich in MN resulted in Parkinsonism or any motor disturbances in general. - Included were 115 adults above 40 years of age of either sex and resident in a rural area of Southern Schleswig-Holstein with a continuous well-water supply of at least 10 years. MN content of well-water had been continuously monitored in all wells for at least six years prior to this investigation. Two proband groups were studied: group A (74 probands; mean age 56.9 +/- 11.8 yrs.) had a MN content of well-water of equal or less than 0.05 mg/l, while in group B (41 probands; mean age 57.5 +/- 10.3 yrs.) MN content of well-water was 0.3 mg/l and above. Both groups were matched for sex, nutritional habits and drug intake. Each proband was evaluated for subjective complaints with a standardized symptom list and for motor abilities using the "Motorische Leistungsserie" of Schoppe. Clinical examination used quantified rating scales for anterior horn dysfunction, cerebellar disease, and dystonia. Parkinsonism was evaluated with the Columbia University Rating Scale. - No significant differences emerged, when item values of the symptom list, ratings of any neurological scale (Mann-Whitney´s U-test) and of any subtest of the Schoppe motor abilities (Student´s t-test) were compared. - The study indicates that for equal periods of exposure neither chronic intake of well-water itself, nor differences in the MN concentrations studied contribute to motor deficits whatsoever in exposed probands.

142

Clinical and Genetic Analysis of Neurofibromatosis Typ 2

Mautner V.-F.*, Tatagiba M.°, Laute S., Hazim W., Gottesleben A.*, Schneider E., Samii M.°, Pulst S.M.

* Neurologic Department, Krankenhaus Ochsenzoll, Langenhorner Chaussee 560, 2000 Hamburg 62

° Neurosurgical Department, Nordstadt Krankenhaus, Haltenhoffstr. 41, 3000 Hannover 1

The neurofibromatoses are among the most common inherited disorders of the nervous system and are the most common cause of inherited tumors of the nervous system. Two types can be distinguished on clinical and genetic grounds. Von Recklinghausen neurofibromatosis (NF1) is located on human chromosome 17, the gene for bilateral acoustic neurofibromatosis (NF2) on chromosome 22.

Objektive:
The clinical phenotype of NF2 has only been defined in a few families. We now present the findings in the initial 28 individuals with NF 2. To determine clinical, neuro-radiologic and ocular manifestations of NF2.

Methods:
Ascertainment through patient initiated contacts with the German von Recklinghausen Gesellschaft and response from university neurosurgical departments in the Western states of the Federal Republic of Germany.

Evaluation: All patients received a complete physical examination, slit lamp examination of the eye, and MRI of the brain and spine with gadolinium enhancement. The reported cases represent the first 31 cases that have been evaluated completely. The total study population comprises more than 100 cases with suspected NF2 or multiple tumors of the nervous system.

31 index cases presented with either:

- bilateral acoustic neuromas
- unilateral acoustic neuroma at age < 30.
- multiple CNS tumors
- CNS tumor plus juvenile cataract
- multiple skin tumors without CAL spots

Of these, 28 met the NIH criteria for NF2.

Results:
Eight cases had one or more family members with NF 2. The largest NF2 family had 5 affecteds in 4 generations. Presenting tumors: Acoustic schwannomas in 12 patients, spinal tumors in 3, meningiomas in 3, peripheral neurinomas in 8. The youngest affected individual was symptomatic at 4 years of age with multiple spinal tumors.
MRI detected asymptomatic spinal or acoustic in approximately half the cases. Twelve patients had posterior cataracts, one hat < 5 Lisch nodules.

Conclusions:
NF2 may present with tumors other than acoustic schwannomas. Asymptomatic spinal and acoustic tumors and cataracts are frequent. One third of NF2 cases have a positive family history. MRI of the brain and spine at an early age is recommended for children of NF2 patients.

References:
Wertelecki W, Rouleau GA, Superneau DW et. al. 1988 Neurofibromatosis 2:
Clinical and DNA linkage of a large kindred. N engl J Med; 319: 278-283.

143

THE INCIDENCE OF CEREBROVASCULAR ACCIDENTS IN ASSOCIATION WITH METEOROLOGIC FACTORS

P. Kreitsch, L. Harms and H. W. Kölmel

Department of Neurology, Humboldt-University, Charité Berlin, Germany

INTRODUCTION: Seasonal variation in the incidence of cerebrovascular accidents has been reported in many countries including the United States, Japan, the United Kingdom and Australia. A uniform distribution with peaks in winter-spring and a trough in the summer-autumn related to air temperature has been observed. Contrary reports are from Yugoslavia and Mexico which have not found seasonality in the incidence of cerebrovascular diseases.

METHODS AND MATERIAL: In the present study the incidence of cerebrovascular accidents in association with meteorologic factors was investigated. During an 8-year period from 1981-1988 564 cases of cerebrovascular diseases were treated in the Charité of Berlin, Germany, of which 230 were classified as subarachnoid hemorrhage, 174 as intracerebral (nontraumatic) hemorrhage and 160 as cerebral infarction.

The number of daily cerebrovascular accidents was compared with the following meteorologic parameters: air temperature, relative humidity, watersteam pressure, global radiation and the weather-phases. For all meteorologic factors, excepting the weather-phases, so called character values were used. Character values (-2, -1, 0, 1, 2) estimate, for example, whether the air temperature of a specific day in association to the historical mean is normal, over- or undernormal or even strongly over- or undernormal. The use of character values takes into consideration natural saisonal sways of the climate and therefore also changing adaptations and sensations of the organism. 15°C for example feel different in autumn than in winter.

The weather is definable into 10 weather-phases which include several meteorologic conditions, among them the temperature-humidity environment.

Significance of the correlated variables was tested by means of standard statistical methods, especially Kendall's tau-b.

RESULTS: In the present study a significant saisonal pattern was not observed but characteristical peaks of incidence occurred in April and November which are mainly influenced by the incidence of subarachnoid hemorrhage. The incidence of subarachnoid hemorrhage was negatively correlated with the character values of watersteam pressure and temperature (p<0.05). The incidences of intracerebral hemorrhage and cerebral infarction were not significantly correlated with the investigated meteorologic factors in this study. However, in addition to all cases of cerebrovascular accidents the above mentioned significant correlation with watersteam pressure and temperature was found. Further the weather on the days before and after cerebrovascular accidents was examined and correlated to the days of onset but no significant difference was observed. In the same way monthly differences in weather character were investigated but no different pattern was found which could explain the saisonal peaks of incidence.

DISCUSSION: The frequently reported negative association of cerebrovascular accidents with ambient temperature only means that at the time of incidence peaks in winter-spring the air temperature is low. By use of character values the temperature feeling is concerned. However, a significant association of onset of cerebrovascular accidents with "cold" days relatively to the historical mean was found. But the weather is a complex of various atmospheric changes and affects the human organism as a whole. It cannot be true that one meteorologic factor alone such as the temperature affects the organism. The weather-phases characterize the weather conditions best. Therefore a characteristic pattern of them on the days with cerebrovascular accidents was to be expected but the distribution was found to be homogeneous.

Concerning the last fact the present study does not suggest an association of cerebrovascular accidents with the weather. Only the characteristic saisonal variation of cerebrovascular accidents needs further explanation.

144

Brain imaging: an aid for early detection of brain damage in boxers

A prospective study in amateur boxers using MRI

Holzgraefe, M[1], Lemme, W[1], Funke, W[1] Felix, R[2], Felten, M[3]

1) Neurological University Clinic Göttingen,
2) Dept. of Radiology Free University Berlin,
3) Institut of Sport science Cologne, Germany

Boxing is a sport subject to controversial discussion. Some 80 research papers dealing with the many facets of this subject were published between 1986 and 1988. The majority of these articles indicate that boxing is a dangerous sport. The significance and possible extent of structural damage to the central nervous system (CNS) due to boxing are investigated. Although the diagnosis of acute injuries of the CNS is easily possible with modern imaging methods, detection of slowly evolving cerebral disturbances is more difficult. Beginning with imaging techniques such as pneumo encephalogram and further developed with computed tomography and the high resolution of magnetic resonance imaging (MRI), it has become possible to demonstrate structural changes in the CNS of boxers. Bleeding, especially microhematomas, are considered to be one probable cause of the chronic encephalopathy by boxers. In a prospective study, 13 amateur boxers were investigated with the help of MRI several times before and after their bouts. The MRI investigations were accompanied by neurologic examinations before and after the fights. Among the 13 boxers, 5 demonstrated focal neurological signs following the bouts, without evidence of microhematoma or other structural alterations. The number of head punches did not correlate with the occurence of neurologic signs. In the context of these results the significance of imaging methods is cricital in the evaluation of the development of chronic encephalopathy.

To date, psychological test methods seem to offer the only dependable method in observing the development and potential risk of a dementia pugilistica. Prospective studies alone will be able to define the potential health risk incurred by amateur boxers.

145

Parkinson´s Disease in Twins - the question of genetic risk

P. Vieregge (1), K.A. Schiffke (1), H.-J. Friedrich (2); H. Westphal (3), H.P. Ludin (4), B. Müller (5)
(1) Klinik für Neurologie und (2) Institut für Medizinische Statistik und Dokumentation, Medizinische Universität D-2400 Lübeck; (3) Institut für Immunologie, Christian-Albrechts-Universität D-2300 Kiel; (4) Neurologische Klinik, Kantonsspital CH-9007 St. Gallen; (5) Abteilung für Pädiatrische Genetik, Ludwig-Maximilians-Universität D-8000 München; Federal Republic of Germany and Switzerland.

In an ongoing study on Parkinson´s disease (PD) in twins from Germany and Switzerland 3 out of 9 monozygotic twins pairs (MZ) and 3 of 12 dizygotic twin pairs (DZ) were concordant for PD or Parkinson-associated dementia. Initial symptoms, their lateralization and the predominant clinical expression were remarkably similar among the concordant pairs. At various diagnostic levels no statistical difference emerged between MZ and DZ concordance rates. MZ concordance rate was different from expected rates of population prevalence only for the diagnostic level of Parkinson-associated dementia ($p<0.05$). Frequency of PD and dementia, but not essential tremor, was higher in DZ than in MZ families compared to expected rates from population prevalence. Using the multifactorial-threshold model, the heritability of "liability" was low (0.12). Comparison between MZ and DZ and between affected and unaffected twins gave no differences in mean family size, mean parental age at birth, in birth size and order, or in complications during gestation and birth and congenital abnormalities. Affected twins reported lower birth weight more frequently than their unaffected twins ($p<0.05$). No evidence of predominant maternal transmission across generations could be established. - The contribution of genetic factors in PD etiology is not ruled out. Pedigree analysis renders mitochondrial inheritance unlikely. The association of pre- or perinatal risk factors with discordant disease affliction in twins remains questionable.

146

TREATED PHENYLKETONURIA: DIETARY CONTROL, VEP, AND MRI FINDINGS
Ludolph, A.C., Bick, U.*, Masur, H., Ullrich, K.#
Department of Neurology, Radiology (*), and Pediatrics (#), University of Münster, FRG

In hyperphenylalaninemia (HPA), the reduced activity of the liver enzyme phenylalanine hydroxylase leads to accumulation of phenylalanine. Early dietary restriction of phenylalanine largely prevents neurological deficits in affected patients. However, the consequences of discontinuation of diet in adulthood are unknown. We have studied 22 adult treated patients with hyperphenylalaninemia in order to define their clinical status and to detect possible subclinical defects with the aid of the techniques of visual evoked potentials (VEP) and magnetic resonance imaging (MRI).
Our studies gave clear-cut evidence for neurophysiological and -radiological alterations even in clinically normal patients. However, the presence of subtle neuropsychological deficits seems to be likely and is presently subject to detailed examinations. 38 % of our patients had prolongations of VEP latencies. All type I and type II patients (classical or mild hyperphenylalaninemia, respectively) showed white matter abnormalities on MRI. Changes were most prominent in the posterior periventricular region but also involved the frontal and subcortical white matter in severely affected patients. Type III patients (persistent hyperphenylalaninemia) had only very discrete MRI changes which can probably not be distinguished from findings in controls. The relation of VEP changes and MRI abnormalities to the documented history of dietary control (phenylalanine plasma levels) was not always consistent. Also, the severity of MRI alterations was not always related to the extent of prolongation of VEP latencies. After strict dietary control for 3 months, repeat MRI examinations revealed that the periventricular abnormalities partly regressed but increased again after dicontinuation of strict control. T2-relaxometry (N = 7) showed a biexponential behaviour of T2 in the affected white matter, with a slow component of about 200-450 msec, indicating that periventricular edema may partly cause the changes. H1 spectra obtained in the parietooccipital periventricular white matter (N = 4) showed no grossly abnormal result (NAA, Cr) which indicates the possible absence of major irreversible neuronal damage.
The detailed pathogenesis of the acute reversible and chronic irreversible neurological changes in treated and untreated patients with phenylketonuria is still unknown. However, in contrast to previous opinions the present results clearly indicate that patients with hyperphenylalaninemia should remain on a strict diet during adulthood.

References:
1. Thompson AJ, Smith I, Brenton D, et al. (1990) Lancet ii: 602-605.
2. Bick U, Fahrendorf G, Ludolph AC, Ullrich K (1989) Proc Symposium SSIEM, Munich, abstr p023.
3. Bick U, Fahrendorf G, Ludolph AC, et al. (1991) Eur J Pediatr 150: 185-189.
4. Ludolph AC, Ullrich K, Nedjat S, et al. () Acta Neurol Scand, in press.

147

TOXIC EFFECTS OF 2,3,7,8-TETRACHLORODIBENZO-P-DIOXIN (TCDD) ON THE PERIPHERAL NERVOUS SYSTEM (PNS) OF THE RAT.

F. Grahmann, H. Grehl, D. Claus, B. Neundörfer.

Neurologische Universitätsklinik, D-8520 Erlangen, Germany.

TCDD is an extremely toxic environmental health hazard for humans and animals causing multiple biological effects, but its neurotoxicity is largely unknown and a matter of controversy. The few clinical reports on exposed humans are contradictory and are mostly based on retrospective analyses of exposed persons after industrial accidents (1). Since human exposure has often been to mixtures and TCDD analysis by mass spectroscopy is very costly and technically difficult, there are virtually no quantitative data on neurotoxicity. Whereas some authors report up to 96% toxic polyneuropathies (2), others could not confirm any neurotoxicity at all (3). Animal experiments have not been done so far.

Therefore, we studied the effect of low TCDD doses on the PNS of the rat. 60 adult, male Han/Wistar rats were injected with a single, intraperitoneal dose of 8.8 (group 1), 6.6 (group 2), 4.4 (group 3) or 2.2 (group 4) ug TCDD/kg body weight while the 20 controls received the solvent corn oil only. Wistar rats were chosen because this strain is rather resistant to TCDD while exhibiting most of its toxic effects except mortality. The typical "wasting syndrome" of high-dose TCDD intoxication was not observed. Temperature-controlled, orthodromic nerve conduction velocity studies were performed in pentobarbital anesthesia (50 mg/kg) before the injection, after maximally 6 and after 10 months. By then, there was statistically significant (ANOVA : Fisher-test; Scheffe-F-test), dose-dependent slowing of motor nerve conduction velocity (MCV) of the right sciatic nerve of TCDD-groups 1 and 2 (8.8 and 6.6 ug/kg TCDD) vs. controls and of sensory nerve conduction velocity (SCV) of all TCDD-groups (1-4) vs. controls. Looking at MCV and SCV in a longitudinal section over a period of approximately 10 months, there was significant slowing within each TCDD-group, but not within the controls. At the end of the experiment, pathologic spontaneous activity was observed in the EMG of peripheral muscles (flexor digitorum and tail muscles) in TCDD-group 1 (100%), 2 (93%), 3 and 4 (87% each) and significantly less in the controls (21%). Histologically, semithin sections of the sciatic nerve showed an acute, proximally accentuated, axonal and demyelinating type neuropathy in the TCDD-groups without significant regeneration. Besides acute axonal degeneration, onion bulb formations were present indicating chronic de- and remyelination. There were distinct interindividual differences in the severity of nerve affection within the single groups probably due to genetic heterogeneity or differences in the affinity of TCDD to the aromatic hydrocarbone (Ah-) receptor.

The present results give the first evidence for a toxic neuropathy in rats after a single, low dose of TCDD.

References

1. Skene SA, Dewhurst IC, Greenberg M (1989) Polychlorinated dibenzo-p-dioxins and polychlorinated dibenzofurans : The risks to human health. A review. Human Toxicol 8 : 173-203

2. Klawans HL, Wilson RS, Garron DC (1987) Neurologic problems following exposure to 2,3,7,8-tetrachlorodibenzo-p-dioxin (TCDD, Dioxin). In : Jenner P (ed) Neurotoxins and their pharmacological implications. Raven Press, New York

3. Assenato G, Cervino D, Emmett EA, Longo G, Merlo F (1989) Follow-up of subjects who developed chloracne following TCDD exposure at Seveso. Am J Ind Med 16 (2) : 119-125

148

HEPARIN IN ACUTE ISCHEMIC STOKE IN ORDER TO PREVENT THROMBOEMBOLIC REINFARCTION.

GLAHN, J., STRAETEN, V., BUSSE, O.
NEUROLOGISCHE KLINIK , KLINIKUM MINDEN

Anticoagulation is used in embolic stroke to prevent reinfarction. 239 pat. were anticoagulated with heparin. Therapy started averagely 1.4 days after stroke. the PTT should be prolonged to 1.5-2.5 fold of the normal value. 112 pat. (46.9%) suffered an atherothrombotic stroke, 79 pat. (33%) a cardioembolic stroke and 48 pat. (20.1%) an embolism of unknown etiology. The average duration of heparin therapy was 11.7 days.
Results: 5 pat. (4.5%) with an atherothrombotic stroke had a recurrent stroke, 15 pat. (13.4%) a TIA. From the pat. with cardiogenic embolism, 4 pat. (5.1%) had a reinfarction and 3 pat. (3.8%) a TIA. 3 pat. (6.3%) with embolism of unknown etiology suffered a TIA. A fatal ICH occured in 2 pat.(0.8%). A hemorrhagic transformation was in one pat. the reason for deterioration, in another pat. for death. 5 reinfarctions and 14 TIAs occured in the first 72 hours after onset of therapy, the other within the first week.
Discussion: The anticoagulation in acute ischemic stroke is a low risk therapy even in extended infarction. Type and frequency of the ischemic event depends on the different underlying etiology of stroke. TIAs occured more often in atherothrombotic than in cardioembolic stroke. Despite the efficacy of heparin therapy is still controversial, anticoagulation seems to be justified in acute embolic stroke because of the low risk if there is no indication for thrombolysis in the first hours after the event.

149

CEREBRAL HAZARDS AFTER HLM-ASSISTED HEART OPERATIONS

Dietmar Schneider[1], Jörg Berrouschot[1], Armin Wagner[1], Karl-Friedrich Lindenau[2]

Clinic of Neurology[1], Clinic of Cardiovascular Surgery[2], University of Leipzig, State University of Saxony, Germany

Background und Purpose. Despite of decreasing incidence of serious complications after HLM (heart lung machine)-assisted heart operations cerebral hazards remain a source of postoperative morbidity and mortality. The aim of our study was to identify pre-, peri-, and postoperative risk factors for cerebral hazards. Which negative role does the controlled hypotension play during extracorporal circulation ? Are neuroelectrophysiologic examinations (EEG, BSAEP) able to identify patients with increased cerebral risk prior to heart operations ?
Methods. Pre-, peri-, and postoperatively findings of 590 patients were recorded. The patients were electively operated on the heart using the extracorporal circulation at the Centre of Cardiovascular Surgery of Leipzig University from October 1987 to January 1989. EEG and BSAEP records were carried out prior to the operation. Myocardial protection used induced ventricular fibrillation, systemic and local hypothermia, and cardioplegia of Brettschneider. The following parameters were evaluated: - lowest and mean arterial blood pressure before, during, after aortic cross-clamping, duration of hypotension lower than 50 mm Hg, TM 50-index (time x minute below 50) as unit of low-pressure perfusion time, last not least autopsy data. All variables were analysed for significant associations with each clinical outcome category.
Results. 60 (10 %) of the 590 patients suffered from cerebral complications postoperatively. 8 patients had a cerebral coma led to death of all of them. 11 patients suffered from ischemic stroke, 38 had an acute brain syndrome, and 3 of an epileptic seizure. Significant high-risk factors of the postoperative cerebral coma were: - old age, hypertension, diabetes mellitus, prolonged periods of anaesthesia, operation, and bypass, and frequent postoperative bleedings. Significant high-risk factors of the postoperative ischemic stroke were: - NYHA stage 4, frequent postoperative circulatory insufficiency, frequent postoperative dysrhythmia. Significant high-risk factors of the postoperative acute brain syndrome were: - old age, frequent pre- and postoperative dysrhythmia, prolonged time of cross-clamping, frequent prolonged and low hypotension (TM 50-index 1000). However, the prediction of postoperative cerebral hazards was only 73 %.
History of myocardial infarction, smoking, peripheral vascular disease, history of cerebrovascular accident, history of transient ischemic attacks, hyperlipidaemia, adipositas, hyperuricaemia, pathologic EEG and/or BSAEP, number of operated grafts, kind of operated heart valve, duration of controlled hypotension, lowest and average arterial mean pressure during extracorporal circulation, TM 50-index before, during and after aortic cross-clamping, unexpected intraoperative complications, difficulty in terminating bypass, postoperative infections, renal dysfunction, myocardial infarction, pulmonal alterations, gastrointestinal haemorrhage, reoperation did not have any influence on the cerebral complication rate.
Patients with increased risk towards postoperative cerebral hazards could not be found out by preoperative EEG and BSAEP records. 67 (11 %) of the 590 patients had a preoperative pathologic EEG, 33 out of them showed a subcortical dysfunction, 28 had pathologic background activities, 5 patients had a focus pattern and one patient had a seizure pattern. However no difference might to be found according to pathologic EEG preoperatively between patients with/without cerebral hazards postoperatively. All patients were operated despite their preoperative pathologic EEG findings. 346 (75 %) of the 462 in whom brain stem auditory evoked potentials (BSAEP) were led showed a pathologic BSAEP, 206 out of them (45 %) had a central, 97 (21 %) a peripheral alteration, and 43 (9 %) had a combined central and peripheral alteration. However no differences might to be found according to pathologic BSAEP preoperatively between patients with/without cerebral hazards postoperatively. Also by combination of EEG and BSAEP findings no patient with increased cerebral risk could be found.
Conclusions. Up to now neither single factors nor combinations of several factors can predict significantly cerebral hazards after HLM-assisted heart operations. Probably the preoperative assessment of the cerebral vascular system is required. This can be done by stress tests of the cerebral blood flow as e.g. Diamox-TCD or Diamox-HMPAO-SPECT as screening methods of brain ischemia testing prior to cardiovascular operations. Such a study is in work supported by grants from the Bundesministerium für Forschung und Technik.

150

CLINICAL FINDINGS IN 149 PATIENTS WITH LACUNAR SYNDROMES

Dorr, J., Schneider R.

Department of Neurology, Klinikum RWTH Aachen, Germany

In a prospective study lasting 30 months 149 patients with lacunar syndromes were examined.
At the time of the clinical examination in 40 (29%) patients the neurological deficits had already disappeared. In 53 (38%) both sensory and motor deficits, in 51 (34%) pure motor deficits or ataxic hemiparesis and in 5 (3%) pure sensory deficits were found.
CT-scan was performed in all patients to confirm the clinical diagnosis of lacunar infarcts. Four groups were formed: 1.) patients with leuko-araiosis but without lacunes, 2.) patients with lacunar infarcts but without leuko-araiosis, 3.) patients with both leuko-araiosis and lacunar infarcts, 4.) patients with normal findings. CT-scan showed leuko-araiosis in 55 (38%) cases, lacunar infarcts in 18 (12%), both leuko-araiosis and lacunar infarcts in 41 (29%) and normal findings in 28 (20%) cases.
A statistical analysis (Kruskal-Wallis-Test) was performed for all clinical data: ataxia (p=0.039) and dysathria (p=0.037) were more frequent in group 3. Patients with only leuko-araiosis were significantly older when compared to the others.
In all 149 patients risk factors were evaluated. In 128 (90%) cases hypertension, in 73 (51%) hypercholesteremia, in 73 (51%) cigarette smoking, in 51 (36%) high uric acid, in 51 (36%) stroke in family history and in 49 (35%) diabetes were found. On admission an initial hematocrit of 43% or higher was found in 85 (56%) cases. 70 (47%) of all patients were aged 70 or older.
In a subgroup follow-up (59 patients) within one year 10% had had a second stroke and 19% were dead.

Conclusions:

(1.) leuko-araiosis is a phenomenon of the elderly.
(2.) ataxia and dysarthria are clinical indicators for the combination of leuko-araiosis and lacunar infarcts.
(3.) mortality and the risk for recurrent stroke are high.

151

PATHOPHYSIOLOGY OF STROKE IN CAROTID ARTERY STENOSES ASSESSED BY COMPUTED TOMOGRAPHY

Krapf H, Kleiser B, Widder B

Department of Neurology, University of Ulm, FRG

The risk of hemodynamic stroke in high-grade internal carotid artery (ICA) stenoses can be easily estimated by assessing the cerebrovascular reserve capacity. In contrast, there exists no method of investigating the risk of developing thrombembolic strokes in ICA lesions.

Fig.1
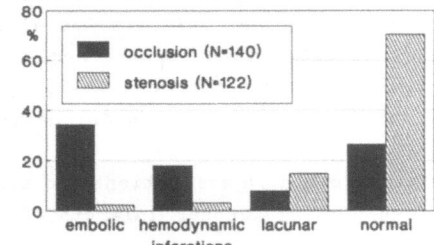

Methods: Of 131 consecutive patients with 140 ICA occlusions and 122 ICA stenoses (65 cases with diameter reductions > 50 %) the hemispheric ischemic lesions in cranial computed tomography (CCT) were analyzed without knowledge of clinical and sonographical findings. The morphological stroke patterns were classified into 3 categories of lacunar, thrombembolic and hemodynamic infarctions.

Results: Ipsilateral to 140 ICA occlusions, 48 thrombembolic, 25 hemodynamic and 11 lacunar infarctions could be identified. In comparison, we found only 3 thrombembolic (p < 0.0001), 4 hemodynamic (p < 0.001) and 18 lacunar lesions (p > 0.05) ipsilateral to 122 ICA stenoses (Fig.1). 43 of the occlusions and 91 of the stenoses showed ipsilaterally negative CCT scans. In total, 19 hemisphares (7.2 %) could not be classified exactly.

Conclusions: Several prospective studies of ICA stenoses indicate a more than 20 % risk of stroke during the developement of an occlusion. Such ischemic events may be due either to periocclusive embolisation or impaired cerebral hemodynamics in cases with insufficient intracranial collateralisation.

In contrast to other CCT studies (3) we found a predominantly thrombembolic nature of strokes in ICA occlusions, confirming the findings of neuropathological investigations (2). Thrombembolic infarctions, however, are well known to be associated with severe neurological deficits and poor clinical prognosis.

In comparison, hemodynamical infarctions in ICA stenoses are rare, and even in ICA occlusions the risk of low-flow infarction is significantly lower than to suffer a thrombembolic stroke. Moreover, cases with critically impaired cerebral hemodynamics can be identified by measuring CO_2 or Diamox reactivity. In our series we found a close correlation between the presence of hemodynamically induced infarctions in the subcortical terminal supply area or watershed zone and an exhausted CO_2 reactivity (1). After carotid surgery an improvement of CO_2 reactivity in all cases with initially impaired cerebral hemodynamics could be demostrated (4).

In summary, our results support the hypothesis of a significantly increased risk of thrombembolic stroke in carotid artery stenoses developing an occlusion. Therefore in progressive, high-grade ICA stenoses carotid surgery may be beneficial even in asymptomatic cases.

References

1. Kleiser B et al. (1991), J Neurol 238: 392-394
2. Landolt AM et al. (1970), Stroke 1: 52-62
3. Ringelstein EB et al. (1983), Stroke 14: 867-875
4. Widder B et al. (1986), Eur Arch Psychatry Neurol Sci 236: 162-168

152

PREVENTION OF STROKE IN ASYMPTOMATIC CAROTID ARTERY STENOSES : BENEFIT OF SURGERY IN PROGRESSIVE CASES

B.Kleiser, B.Widder, H.Krapf, A.Dürr

Department of Neurology, University of Ulm, FRG

Though the value of thrombendarterectomy in severe symptomatic internal carotid artery (ICA) stenoses has recently been proven, the therapeutical concept in asymptomatic cases is still controversial.

Methods: In a non-randomised prospective study 143 patients with 179 ICA stenoses with initial diameter reductions of 40-80 % were sonographically and clinically reinvestigated in 6 month intervals. Death, ipsilateral neurological symptoms and occlusion of the vessel were defined as endpoints. Patients with progressive stenoses exceeding 80 % diameter reduction and/or ipsilateral TIA/minor stroke were submitted to carotid thrombendarterectomy. Progression was defined as an increase of at least 2 kHz in systolic Doppler frequency (referred to 4 MHz ultrasound) and/or more than 10 % of diameter reduction measured by duplex scanning.

Results: 127 patients could be followed for a mean period of 46 months. Out of 44 patients with progressive ICA stenoses, 17 developed a diameter reduction of more than 80 %. Of these, 14 underwent thrombendarterectomy, the remaining refused surgery. Another patient was operated because of recent neurological symptoms in a stable stenosis. During the perioperative period, one patient suffered a major stroke. In the postoperative course (mean 12 months) none of them developed neurological symptoms. In the non-operated group of 112 patients, 3 suffered a stroke ipsilateral to a stenosis. All of them showed progression of the stenosis.

Conclusions: Several other studies in the literature report a significantly increased risk of stroke for patients with asymptomatic severe ICA stenoses as compared to lower grade stenoses. In contrast, none of our patients with ICA stenoses of initially ≥ 70 % (N = 52) developed relevant neurological symptoms. All strokes in our group occurred in patients with initially moderate, but progressive stenoses. This indicates the importance of progression as an own risk factor for cerebral ischemia. In consequence, further surgical trials in asymptomatic patients should deal not only with severe, but also with moderate, rapidly progressive ICA stenoses.

153

Prognostic and therapeutic relevance of circadian blood pressure variations after cerebral infarction

D. Sander and J. Klingelhöfer

Department of Neurology, Technical University of Munich, Möhlstraße 28, W-8000 München 80

Several epidemiological studies indicate hypertension as the primary risk factor for the development of cerebral infarction. In contrast the knowledge about the significance of circadian blood pressure variations after cerebral infarction is limited. The objective of our study was to analyse the alterations in circadian blood pressure patterns after cerebral infarction and to establish their possibe prognostic and therapeutic relevance.

For this purpose, a non-invasive 24h blood-pressure measurement was carried out repeatedly during the clinical course in 22 patients with cerebral infarction of various pathogenesis. The blood pressure was measured with a portable oscillometric monitoring system (Spacelabs ABD-Monitor 90207). Measurements were performed for 24 hours at intervals of 15 minutes.

Depending on the pathogenesis of the infarction, different alterations of circadian blood pressure profiles could be observed: patients with severe stenosis or occlusion of the internal carotid artery and hemodynamic infarction frequently showed an increased amplitude of circadian blood pressure fluctuations with hypotensive values at night. Compared to a control population, the range of variation between day and night values, which was over 40% in occasional cases, was significantly raised (p<0.05). In patients with distinct daytime hypertension and additional inadequate collateralisation capacity of the circle of Willis (vasomotor reactivity less than 40% after CO_2 stimulation), a prolonged break down of the blood-brain barrier could be observed. Administration of an ACE inhibitor (5-10mg enalapril) in the morning led to a reduction of the hypertensive daytime values with largely unchanged nighttime blood pressure. This normalization of the circadian blood pressure variability was accompanied by clinical improvement and recovery of the blood-brain barrier. In contrast to this, patients with thrombembolic territorial infarctions showed a substantially reduced amplitude of circadian blood pressure fluctuations in the initial phase. In these patients, even if initially normotensive, the physiological nocturnal blood pressure decrease was clearly reduced or absent. In the further clinical course a normalisation of the circadian blood pressure variability frequently ocurred even without antihypertensive therapy. Patients with the most pronounced reduction of blood pressure variability showed an extensive infarction of the middle cerebral artery territory, including the insula region.

The constellation of hemodynamic cerebral infarction, severe obstruction of an brain supplying artery and increased amplitude of circadian blood pressure fluctuations can lead to a prolonged break down of blood-brain barrier. In patients with recurrent cerebral ischemia, an altered circadian blood pressure pattern should be considered in the differential diagnosis. For this reason, additional recording of the circadian blood pressure patterns may be of prognostic and therapeutic relevance.

154

Lipoidgranulomatosis Erdheim Chester (LEC), neurological signs and symptoms

J.Martin, K.Schimrigk, C.Kujat, H.Lehmann*
Univ. of Saarland, Dep. of Neurology and Neuroradiology, D-6650 Homburg,
*Evang. Krankenhaus, D-6660 Zweibrücken

In 1931 W. Chester(1) described two patients with lipoidgranulomas in the long bones excluding the epiphyseal regions. For 60 years 30 patients have been described with the characteristic infiltration of the long bones. Histologically foamy lipid laden histiocytes with S-100 protein are found similar to histiocytosis X. The clinical findings correspond to the extraosseal organs involved: lung, cutis, kidney, orbita, heart, retroperitoneal space and brain. The patient we present has suffered from a temporary diabetes insipidus, an arterial hypertension developes accompagnied by an elevated blood sedimentation rate. One year later an "idiopathic", peripheral paresis of the facial nerve and furthermore a dysarthria and ataxia appear. A cutaneous lipoidgranulomatosis develops in the face excluding the periocular and perioral regions. The left kidney has to be removed because of a stenosis of the renal artery, a coronary artery disease is clinically evident and treated by angioplasty, a pericardial effusion requires a pericardiocentesis. The x-ray of the chest reveals an interstitial fibrosis of the lung, an aneurysm of the abdominal aorta and an occlusion of a femoral artery requires surgical intervention. The MRI of the skull shows signal intensive lesions in the region of pons and mesencephalon, there is a tumor of the left choroid plexus storing Gd-DTPA for more than two weeks, a phenomenom already described in a dural manifestation(2). The right internal carotid artery is occluded while the left one has a stenosis of fifty percent. It is remarkable that almost all vessels (i.e. coronary, renal, femoral, extracranial arteries) are narrowed by sclerotic lesions. The reason of the generalized atherosclerosis is unknown. Beside vascular risk factors (i.e. hypertension, hyperfibrinogenemia, elevated lipoprotein a, but not elevated cholesterol) parameters of inflammation (i.e. blood sedimentation rate, C-reactive protein) are elevated. After treatment with methylprednisone a normalization of these parameters is achieved. Thus we conclude that an immunsuppressive treatment might have a beneficial effect and reduces inflammatory activity. Because of the various signs and symptoms LEC should be considered in the differential diagnosis of both inflammatory and ischemic neurological diseases.

References:
1. Chester W (1931) Über Lipoidgranulomatose. Virchows Arch (A) 279:561-602
2. Tien RD, Brasch RC, Jackson DE, Dillon WP (1989) Cerebral Erdhein- Chester disease: persistent enhancement with Gd- enhancement on MR- images. Radiology 172: 791-792

155

B. HOFFERBERTH

Neurologische Abteilung, Krankenhaus Lindenbrunn,
D-3256 Coppenbrügge

The Training of Saccadic Eye Movements in Patients with Unilateral Stroke

Strokes in the region supplied with blood via the middle cerebral artery do not only lead to contralateral hemiparesis, but frequently also affect oculomotor activity and lead to horizontal pareses of gaze movement. The damage may affect the frontal eye field or the frontopontine tract, mostly in the internal capsule. In the initial stage, this leads to the familiar turning of gaze and frequently also turning of the head to the diseased side (déviation conjugée). In the course of rehabilitation, there is marked slowing of the horizontal saccades to the healthy side. For the patient, this slowing of unilateral horizontal eye movements entails greater difficulty in reading and an impendiment of optically based spatial orientation.

In 100 patients with unilateral stroke of the cerebral media artery, a daily systematic saccade training was carried out for at least 30 days after occurence of the stroke. For this purpose, a battery - powered strip fitted with LEDs was used. This simple stimulation instrument is mobile and could be used everywhere in the hospital. A group of 100 patients with unilateral stroke who were not subjected to saccade training served as a reference group.

The recording and the computer-supported evaluation of the horizontal saccades using electrooculo-graphy, determination of the speed of reading and a questionaire on spatial orientation served as weekly control parameters.

Compared to the control population, a marked improvement of the horizontal saccades to the side contralateral to the stroke was observed as a result of the saccade training in the patient population. This was accompanied by an increase of the reading speed and an improvement of spatial orientation. Regular and timely performance of horizontal saccade training is to be recommended in patients with unilateral media stroke.

156

IMPROVEMENT OF COGNITIVE FUNCTIONS AFTER SAB AND ANEURYSM SURGERY BY THE GINKGO-BILOBA-SPECIAL-EXTRACT LI 1370

K. Maier-Hauff, D. Laudahn
Department of Neurosurgery, UKRV, FU Berlin,
Augustenburger Platz 1, 1000 Berlin 65, Germany

Introduction

Subarachnoid hemorrhage from a ruptured aneurysm often results not only in neurological deficits, but also in important cognitive irritations in spite of a favorable spontaneous and operative development (2).

Methods

In a placebo-controlled, double-blind trial the effectiveness of the Ginkgo-biloba-special-extract LI 1370 should be examined. After written agreement of an ethical commission the study was performed in 50 ambulant patients. The follow-up examination period after surgery was 7 - 42 months. The post-operative clinical judgement was made following the Glasgow-Outcome-Coma-Scale. The neuropsychological test battery contained the examination of attention with the Zimmermann-Test-Battery, Freiburg as well as the examination of the short term memory on verbal and non-verbal level. Duration: 12 weeks. Dosage: 3 x 50 mg Ginkgo-biloba-special-extract LI 1370 (Kaveri®, Lichtwer Pharma GmbH) or placebo. The control examinations were made in week 0, 6 and 12.

Results

The study showed in the field of attention a significant reduction of reaction time within the active treatment group. Also in parts of the short term memory as repeating of figures a significant improvement by 65 % appeared in the active treatment group compared to 2 % in the placebo group. No improvements were seen in the field of the spatial oriented abilities of the patients.

Summary

The study showed that cognitive disturbances in patients after SAB and aneurysm surgery can be influenced positively with the Ginkgo-biloba-special-extract LI 1370. Since an improvement of blood flow rather plays a minor role for injuries after SAB and aneurysm surgery, the Ginkgo-biloba-special-extract seems to influence the metabolism of the tissue positively. Several mechanisms are responsible for the effectiveness of Ginkgo-biloba-extracts, as e. g. effects on blood circulation, rheological effects (antagonistic to platelet activating factor receptors, decreased viscosity) and metabolic changes (1). As to the results of this study the metabolic effect is of most importance, since vasospasmus or circulatory changes were no longer of importance by the time of examination. In conclusion: In patients after SAH and aneurysm surgery the drug treatment should be started early to improve the cognitive disfunction in this patients.

References

1. Drieu K (1985) Multiplicity of effects of Ginkgo biloba extract: currents status and new trends. In: Effects of Ginkgo Biloba Extract on Organic Cerebral Impairment. A. Agnoli, J.R. Rapin, V. Scapagnini, W.V. Weitbrecht. John Libbey Eurotext Ltd.

2. Ljunggren B et al. (1985) Cognitive impairment and admustment in patients without neurological deficits after aneurysmal SAH. J Neurosurg 62: 673 - 679.

157

Reasons for failure of anti-toxoplasma prophylaxis in AIDS-patients

J. Madlener[1], W. Enzensberger[1], P. Herdt[1], P. Kalus[1], E.B. Helm[2], P.-A. Fischer[1]

[1]Department of Neurology
[2]Department of Infectious Diseases
University Hospital, Frankfurt/Main, Germany

Objective:

Toxoplasmic encephalitis is the most frequent cause of focal intracerebral lesions in patients with AIDS. CNS toxoplasmosis develops as a result of local reactivation of an earlier acquired latent toxoplasmic brain infection. HIV-patients who meet the diagnostic criteria of toxoplasmic encephalitis are usually empirically treated with pyrimethamine and sulfonamides. The diagnosis is confirmed by a clinical response to the treatment within 1 - 2 weeks and a clear radiographic remission (CT / MRI) within 2 - 3 weeks. Anti-toxoplasma drugs available to date are only effective against replicating Toxoplasma gondii tachyzoits, but not against the cyst form. After clinical remission those cysts remain a source of reactivation of acute toxoplasmic encephalitis. This is the reason, why lifelong prophylactic therapy is recommended after successful treatment of acute encephalitis. We use 50 mg pyrimethamine daily and 15 mg folinic acid twice a week. It was the aim of our study to analyse the reasons of failure of anti-toxoplasma prophylaxis.

Methods:

We evaluated 21 AIDS-patients with successfully treated toxoplasmic encephalitis retrospectively, as documented by clinical and CT scan response who suffered a relapse. Relapses were diagnosed when the typical combination of clinical signs and symptoms and CT / MRI findings were seen after a period of remission.

Results:

The rate of relapses in our patients was 23% (21/93). In most cases a probable reason for the failure of the prophylaxis was found:

9x   cessation of prophylactic therapy
2x   low prophylactic dosage (< 50 mg pyrimethamine daily)
6x   drug interaction with concomitant medication (4x anticonvulsants, 1x tuberculostatics, 1x both)
2x   anticonvulsants plus low prophylactic medication (< 50 pyrimethamine daily)
2x   unknown

The average CD4 lymphocyte count in patients with relapse of toxoplasmic encephalitis was 7/μl (range 0 - 22).

Conclusions:

Our data show, that CNS toxoplasmosis was reactivated because of either cessation of chemotherapy prophylaxis by the patient himself or by his physician or insufficient dosing or drug interactions. We therefore propose a regular control of the patient's compliance and higher dosing of pyrimethamine, if the patient takes other medication known to interact with pyrimethamine such as anticonvulsants.

158

Changes of cerebral hemodynamics in sleep apnea as a cerebrovascular risk factor

J. Klingelhöfer[1], G. Hajak[2], D. Sander[1], M. Schulz-Varszegi[2], E. Rüther[2], B. Conrad[1]

[1]Department of Neurology, Technical University of Munich, Möhlstraße 28, W-8000 München 80; [2]Department of Psychiatry, University of Göttingen, von-Siebold-Straße 4, W-3400 Göttingen, Germany

A correlation between habitual snoring, sleep apnea and increased risk of myocardial infarction is under discussion. However, there are very few systematic investigations of cerebral hemodynamics and CO_2 reactivity in altered alveolar ventilation. In order to investigate the effect of nocturnal apneic episodes on the flow parameters in the middle cerebral artery, about 1000 apneic episodes were analysed.

A pulsed Doppler system (2 MHz) was used for continuous overnight recordings of intracranial flow patterns together with simultaneous polysomnography, continuous blood pressure recordings, and measurements of endexpiratory CO_2. The CO_2 reactivity during the apneic episodes was defined as the ratio of the percentage mean flow velocity increase at the difference between endexpiratory CO_2 measurements before and after the respective apneic episodes.

There was an even rise of mean flow velocity by a 19% to 219% in each stage of sleep during the apneic episodes with a maximum in the REM sleep. With recommencement of breathing, the mean flow velocity rapidly fell to the initial value. The rise in blood pressure varied between 12.5% and 83.1% within one apneic episode. In the waking state, CO_2 reactivity was in a normal range (4.4% ± 1.2%). In the sleep stages 1 and 2 was a pronounced rise of CO_2 reactivity ($p < 0.005$ compared to awake values). The greatest increase was found in REM sleep with a rise of CO_2 reactivity up to three times the waking value ($p < 0.0001$ compared to sleep stage 2).

The changes of mean flow velocity could be interpreted as reactive adaptation processes because of CO_2 and blood pressure increase corresponding to the apnea. The increased CO_2 reactivity during sleep may indicate a "hypersensitivity" of intracranial vascular CO_2 or pH receptors and a disturbance of central catecholaminergic and cholinergic systems. The cerebral hemodynamics accompanying the altered nocturnal alveolar ventilation is a possible risk factor for the occurence of cerebral ischemia: 1. Owing to the raise of CO_2 reactivity during sleep, the alterations in CO_2 associated with the apneic episodes lead to pronounced blood flow velocity fluctuations in the cerebral arteries. It can be assumed that the alterations of the vessel wall tension resulting from the flow velocity fluctuations lead to a chronic strain on the brain vessels with consequent micro- and macroangiopathies. 2. Rises of blood pressure level depending on the respective sleep stage were found in patients who showed normotensive or only slightly hypertensive blood pressure values during the day. 3. Under certain conditions the complex hemodynamic changes in sleep and the substantially reduced blood flow velocity in the early morning hours might lead to a critical reduction in cerebral perfusion resulting in an ischemia. This is consistent with the high rate of cerebral infarctions at this time.

159

CLINICAL VARIABILITY OF TRANSMISSIBLE VIRUS DEMENTIA (CREUTZFELDT-JAKOB-DISEASE) AND PRECAUTIONS IN MEDICAL CARE

Dr. J. Braun[1] , Prof. Dr. H. Glasner[1] , Prof. Dr. J. Cervos-Navarro[2]

1 Neurologische Abteilung Krankenhaus Neukölln , Berlin
2 Institut für Neuropathologie , FU Berlin

Objective and background. In three case reports we describe the clinical variability of C-J-D , comparing with CCT , MRI , CSF , and EEG. Since the disease is transmissible and letal we recommend in unclear, suspected cases a biopsy during lifetime to confirm diagnosis and take precautions.

Methods and results. During the last five years we saw three verified cases of C-J-D , which is a three times higher rate as worldwide. Case 1. A 55-year-old women presented,after a five month period of vertigo and progressive gait disorder, ataxia, dysarthria, and first signs of dementia. The symptoms progressed rapidly to coma and death one month later. EEG showed only in the final stadium global changings, CSF was normal without intrathecal immunoreaction. MRI lesions were found in basal ganglia, cerebral cortex and cerebral white matter. Histopathological findings were a neuronal loss, and foci of a status spongiosis in the cerebral cortex and a moderate proliferation of astrocyts.

Case 2. A 65-year-old man presented with progressive gait disorder and nightly myoclonus. Only a few months later he developed cranial nerve lesions, progressive dementia and severe ataxia ,unable to walk , akinetic mutism, dying two months later. EEG revealed both-sided theta-delta slowing , CCT and MRI without abnormalities, CSF was normal . Histopathological changes were found only in the thalamus and the basal ganglia. This is a rare form of C-J-D , known as Stern-Gracin-typ.

Case 3. A 45-year-old man presented, after a three month period of depression , with aphasia, upper and lower motor-neuron signs, myoclonus and confusion. During the following two month dementia appeared and progressed rapidly to coma.CSF and all serum chemistries were normal. CCT without pathological findings. EEG showed rhythmic bi- and triphasic steep waves , MRI found microlesions in basal ganglia and cerebral white matter. The diagnosis was confirmed by biopsy during life and showed the typical changings.

Conclusions. An early onset of dementia in combination with neurological disorder, especially myoclonus, negative CSF and specific changings in EEG and MRI is suspected as C-J-D. In cases of a rapidly progress we recommend a biopsy during life, as the only possibility to confirm diagnosis of C-J-D.

To get exact epidemiological data we demand autopsy of all patients who showed sings of dementia and an initiation of an obligatory reporting in verified cases of C-J-D.

A patient`s blood , CSF, nerve and cerebral tissues shoud be considered a potential source of infection, but there is no evidence that stool, urine salvia and other secretions are infectious. All instruments that have come into direct contact with blood or tissues of patients with unknown dementia shoud be autoclaved for one hour by 132° C or immersed in 5% sodium hypochlorite for two hours.For EEG and EMG examinations on demented patients we recommend to use surface electrodes and after using a desinfection with 5% sodium hypochlorite solution. Surgical instruments and ophthalmological tonometers should be autoclaved or immersed in the same way.No demented or confused patient shoud be accepted as blood donor or organ donor for transplantation. An unusual risk of C-J-D exist not for medical workers except for pathologists and neurosurgists, although precautions are necessary in all patients who had evidence of dementia associated with neurological disorders.

160

RISK FACTORS IN LUMBAR INTERVERTEBRAL DISK DISEASE AFTER OPERATIVE TREATMENT

Wolfgang A. Dauch and Bernhard L. Bauer
Neurosurgical Department, Philipps University, Marburg, Germany

Intervertebral disk surgery turns out to be successful in about 75 per cent of patients. This number seems to be rather invariable across decades and continents. Thus, one out of every four patients does not make much of a profit from the operation, even when the indication seems to be correct and the operative technique adequate. In this situation, the results of operative treatment could possibly be improved and unsuccessful operations could be avoided if it were possible to identify unpromising patients in advance.

This is a classical goal of clinical risk research. Its methods are well developed now and might be able to predict outcome of treatment in individual cases (albeit in a statistical, not a deterministic manner), taking risk factors into account which have been derived from clinical trials. We performed a meta-analysis of 18 such trials in which the authors tried to find patient-specific risk factors for an unsuccessful outcome after lumbar intervertebral disk surgery. Supplementary, we regard the results of a prospective clinical trial of our own, dealing with follow-up data six months after intervertebral disk surgery in 75 patients.

Results can be summarized as follows:

1) The findings in risk factor analysis are influenced by the way in which the target variable (in this cas: success of operation) is defined.

2) We found 84 variables beeing investigated with respect to their predictive power. Of these, 33 were considerd at least twice:
   - In four factors, the respective authors are agreed on them beeing predictive for an unsuccessful outcome: long duration of sick leave, preoperative unemployment, low intensity of preoperative pain, and hypochondriasis, due for instance to the Minnesota Multiphasic Personality Inventory (MMPI).
   - In some other factors, there is an agreement that they are not predictive: the results of intelligence testing, the male-female-index in the MMPI, and some signs in conventional x-ray imaging.
   - In the majority of factors, however, there is considerable disagreement about their predictive power: for instance age, gender, duration of symptoms, spinal injury, neurological findings, level of operation, education, marital status, and some items of psychological testing.

3) Methodological pitfalls may account for some of these disagreements, for instance occult non-linearity, or interdependencies of risk factors from each other.

In the face of these insufficiencies, we cannot yet provide a reliable predictive algorithm for the results of lumbar intervertebral disk surgery, but the methods of clinical risk research, appropriately applied, seem to be promising tools for this purpose.

Platform session IV
Cerebrospinal fluid analysis
Clinical neurochemistry

161

Antibodies to Purkinje Cells as an Indicator of Therapeutic Efficiency in Paraneoplastic Cerebellitis

E. Stark, U. Patzold[1], U. Wurster
Hannover Medical School, Municipal Hospital Braunschweig[1]

Autoimmune phenomena are of major importance in the pathogenesis of the main paraneoplastic diseases in humans. The autoimmune process is probably triggered by oncogenic antigens, which are cross-reactive or identical with certain neural antigens. Despite the known pathomechanism these syndromes are still considered as non-treatable. We report two cases of paraneoplastic cerebellar degeneration, in which intensive immunosuppression with cytostatics lead to considerable neurological improvement.

In the first patient neurological disease appeared 6 months after the resection of a carcinoma of the oviduct. Two months later the patient was severely disabled. The severe ataxia improved considerably after cyclophosphamid therapy with a concimitant decrease in serum levels and intracerebral synthesis of the autoantibody.

Treatment of the second patient was started much earlier, but after two cycles the therapy was discontinued by the patient. After a clinical relapse the disease was stable for a long period. Although the serum level of the autoantibody remained unchanged, the amount of autoantibody synthesized intracerebrally was significantly decreased.

Despite their low incidence paraneoplastic diseases of the CNS are of particular interest for the investigation of other putative CNS autoimmune diseases. For example, mild immunosuppression has only marginal benefit in multiple sclerosis and intrathecal immunoglobulin G synthesis is hardly affected by this kind of treatment.

In contrast, our patients with paraneoplastic diseases treated with intensive immunosuppression showed a favourable clinical response and a clearcut decrease of local antibody production could be demonstrated.

162

FERRITIN IN CSF: ORIGIN AND CLINICAL RELEVANCE

Wick M.[1], Huber M.[1], Fink W.[1], Einhäupl K.[2], Fateh-Moghadam A.[1]

[1]Institute for Clinical Chemistry and [2]Neurological Department ofKlinikum Großhadern, Munich University, Marchioninistr. 15, D-8000 MÜNCHEN 70, F. R. G.

Whereas an intact blood-CSF-barrier can be expected to enable the passage of only 0.1 % of a 450 kD-protein, ferritin is found in concentrations up to 10 µg/l in normal CSF, slightly elevated in CNS inflammations, infarctions and tumour infiltration (2) and exceeding serum values after subarachnoid hemorrhage (3).

The purpose of the following study was to characterize CSF ferritin and investigate its blood-CSF-barrier dependency to support the hypothesis of a possible production within the CNS. Additionally, CSF cells were to be analyzed as possible sources of CSF ferritin. Since preliminary results had shown the possible clinical value of CSF ferritin for discrimination between genuine CNS hemorrhage and traumatic spinal tap (3), this was to be assessed in a prospective study.

The influence of serum ferritin on CSF ferritin content was determined by ELISA (Enzymun-Test Ferritin, Boehringer Mannheim, F.R.G.) in paired CSF and serum specimens from 367 unselected patients; Ferritin CSF/serum ratios were evaluated against albumin ratio as a barrier indicator according to Reiber's and Felgenhauer's (1) principles. To exclude the possibility of ferritin crossing the barrier as low-molecular-weight subunits, the molecular weight (MW) of CSF ferritin was determined by HPLC gel filtration (HiLoad Superdex 200, Pharmacia, Uppsala Sweden) in 6 patients with high CSF ferritin (>400 ng/ml); isoelectric points (pI) were determined as well by IEF (isoelectric focusing, pH 3.5-9.5, agarose, Multiphor,Pharmacia-LKB, Uppsala, Sweden), and immunoblot with POD-conjugated-anti-ferritin-antiserum (Dakopatts, Glostrup, Denmark). The role of CSF cells as a source of CSF ferritin was analyzed in 21 highly cellular specimens (>100/µl) by indirect immunofluorescence using a polyclonal anti-ferritin antiserum (Dakopatts). Clinical relevance was evaluated in 200 cases clinically suggestive of CNS hemorrhage and/or containing >500 erythrocytes per µl CSF.

We found no correlation between CSF and serum ferritin concentration (R=0.193), no dependency of CSF ferritin from CSF/serum albumin ratio (R = 0.082) and no correlation between CSF/serum ferritin ratio and the albumin ratio (R = 0.114). Furthermore, in 99% of cases, ferritin ratios were by far higher than albumin ratios. MW of CSF ferritin was found at 449 + 8.6 kD; immunoblot after isoelectric focusing showed 6-10 isoferritin bands at a pI 5.0-6.0, corresponding to the properties of "basic" storage ferritins. Very intense ferritin stainings were observed in macrophages after subarachnoid hemorrhage, moderate ones in tumor cells, leukocytes were weakly ferritin positive on membrane surface. The cellular ferritin content, but not the cell count correlated to CSF ferritin concentration in the corresponding diseases.

We conclude that ferritin in CSF is predominantly derived from sources within the CNS itself. Apart from cerebral parenchyma, at least in cases with pleocytosis, CSF cells may produce ferritin. Degradation of erythrocytes by macrophages after subarachnoid hemorrhage yields high amounts of surplus iron, stored as non-toxic basic ferritin, which is released into CSF , thus facilitating the discrimination of genuine hemorrhage and traumatic spinal puncture (3). Data on sensitivity and specificity are provided.

1) Reiber H., Felgenhauer K. (1987) Protein transfer at the blood cerebrospinal fluid barrier and the quantitation of the humoral immune response within the central nervous system; Clin. Chim. Acta 163: 319-328

2) Sindic C. J. M. et al. (1981) The clinical relevance of ferritin concentration in the cerebrospinal fluid; J. Neurol. Neurosurg Psychiatry 44: 329-33

3) Wick et al. (1988) Ferritin in cerebrospinal fluid differentation between central nervous system hemorrhage and traumatic spinal puncture; J. Clin. Pathol. 41: 809

163

NEOPTERIN (NPT), BETA-2 MICROGLOBULIN (B2M) AND TRYPTOPHAN (TRP) IN CSF AND SERUM IN HIV-1 INFECTED INDIVIDUALS.

M. Proescholdt, W. Enzensberger, L. Demisch, P.-A. Fischer
Department of Neurology, University Hospital, Frankfurt/Main, Germany

INTRODUCTION: There is evidence that disease progression in HIV-1-infected patients is not only caused by the decrease of CD4+ T cells, but also by repeated activation of the immune system. Npt and B2M are markers of the cell-mediated immune system. Npt reflects interferon-γ induced activation of monocytes/macrophages. B2M, as a subunit of the major histocompatibility complex (MHC) class I molecule, is expressed on all nucleated cells, especially on activated T lymphocytes. Trp is known to be catabolized through the kynurenine-pathway after interferon-γ induced stimulation of indoleamine-2,3-dioxygenase (IDO) and can therefore serve as an indirect marker. We have evaluated these markers in HIV-1-infected patients to assess their diagnostic value in neuromanifestations.

METHODS: In a prospective study we have analysed cerebrospinal fluid (CSF) and serum samples of 27 individuals without neurological or internal disorders (controls) and of 41 HIV-1-infected patients. According to the Frankfurt staging categories: Stage 1 (early HIV-1 infection): n=3, stage 2a (PGL): n=3, stage 2b (ARC): n=4, stage 3 (AIDS): n=31.
4 of the 41 patients did not have neurological complications (No), 10 showed primary (N1), 14 secondary (N2) and 13 primary and secondary neuromanifestations (N1,2).
Npt was measured by RIA (IMMUtest Neopterin, Henning Berlin GmbH), B2M by MEIA (Abbott-GmbH) and Trp by HPLC.

RESULTS: HIV-1-infected patients showed highly significant increases of Npt and B2M in CSF and serum and a decrease of Trp in comparison to our controls (Kruskal-Wallis- rank-variance analysis). Npt and Trp findings in CSF were independent of blood-brain-barrier impairment, whereas B2M correlated significantly with the albumin-index (r=.4393, p=.005). CSF (but not serum) Npt and B2M showed a significant correlation (r=.4745, p=.001). CSF Trp and Npt did not (r=-.2022, p=.109). CSF Npt, B2M and Trp findings were not predictive for the clinical stage of the HIV-1-infected patients, nor did they differentiate between primary and secondary neuromanifestations. However, patients with acute and/or severe neurological involvement had extremely high (Npt, B2M) and low (Trp) CSF concentrations, respectively, and particularly a high Npt CSF/serum ratio. Also, high CSF Npt levels correlated significantly (r=-.5573, p=.013) with a poor survival.

CONCLUSIONS: Activation of the cell-mediated immune system in the CNS, as reflected by Npt, B2M and Trp, can be seen in all stages of HIV-1 disease. Our data show that such an intrathecal immunological activation may play a crucial role in HIV-1-infected patients with neurological complications. However, Npt, B2M and Trp are non-specific markers and do not allow differentiation between primary and secondary neuromanifestations. On the other hand they are helpful in assessing the acuity and severity of the neurological involvement and should therefore be included in the routine CSF analysis in HIV-1-infected patients.

164

DISCRIMINATION OF HERPES SIMPLEX VIRUS TYPES 1 AND 2 BY MICROPLATE HYBRIDIZATION OF AMPLIFIED DNA SEGMENTS FROM CSF OF PATIENTS WITH HSV ENCEPHALITIS AND MENINGITIS

H.Shoji, R.Hondo*
First Department (Neurology) of Internal Medicine, Kurume University of Medicine, Asahimachi 67, Kurume, Japan, *Department of Microbiology, Institute of National Public Health, Tokyo, Japan

In CNS infections caused by herpes simplex virus (HSV), it is generally accepted that adult acute encephalitis is due to HSV type 1, whereas myelitis and meningitis are produced by HSV type 2. As compromised hosts or atypical HSV CNS infections are increasing, the type is not always uniform. In this study, the common sequences between HSV types 1 and 2 were used as primers for PCR from CSF of 8 patients with probable HSV encephalitis and meningitis, then the amplified DNA segments were differentiated into types 1 and 2 by stringent microplate – hybridization.

Patients and methods : Between 1986 and 1990, 15 CSF samples were obtained from 8 patients with 5 acute encephalitis, 1 brain stem encephalitis and 2 meningitis. 13 CSFs were also taken from 10 control patients such as lumbar disc hernia. All samples were stored at -80 ℃ until applying PCR and hybridization.

The commom primers for HSV types 1 and 2 were those chosen by Sakaoka et al., plus strand, 5' – AGACGTTTGCCTGGTTCCTGG – 3', and minus strand, 5 – 'AGCCGCCACCGCCTGCT – 3'. Biotin – labeled probes for each type were made also by PCR as previously described by Inouye et al. 500 μ l of CSF was ultracentrifuged for 1 h at 28,000 G, followed by phenol – chloroform extraction, ethanol precipitation and then reconstituted to 50 μ l volume buffer. DNA was ampfied according to the protocol of Saiki et al.. The The amplified DNAs were incubated overnight for immobilization on microplate wells. The biotin – labeled probes were added, and the microplates were immersed at 62 ℃ overnight, with is most appropriate temperature for the discrimination in this hybridization.

Results : Six patients were positive, of which 3 HSV type 1 and 3 HSV type 2 were identified, repectively. In 1 case of brain stem encephalitis and 1 case of meningitis, HSV type 1 was detected, although the type of brain stem encephalitis is uncertain and the meningitis is usually produced by type 1. In 1 case of adult acute encephalitis which is regarded as type 1 infection, HSV type 2 was found. Our report indicates that this method is useful for typing of herpes simplex viruses in CNS infection.

165

Diagnosis of neuroborreliosis using serologic tests and DNA amplification

H.W. Kölmel, R. Lange, H. Bocklage

Department of Neurology, Charité, Humboldt University Berlin, Schumannstr. 20/21, 1040 Berlin

Introduction:

Lyme borreliosis is a contagious disease transmitted by ticks of the genus *Ixodes*. Aside from dermatological, cardial and rheumatological manifestations, the multi-systemic disease spectrum also covers affections of the nervous system (neuroborreliosis), which occur in many different shapes and sizes, frequently imitating the clinical symptoms of other diseases. Due to the fact that attempts to culture the pathogen from the cerebrospinal fluid (CSF) of neuroborreliosis have failed, rapid and direct verification has only become possible with the introduction of polymerase chain reaction (PCR). By implementing non-overlapping primer pairs from the flagellin (fla) gene of *B. burgdorferi* we have established a two-stage PCR to identify the pathogen of the Lyme disease. By this method we have managed to detect less than 10 spirochaetes without additional hybridisation. The specificity of the 290bp amplification product could be confirmed by restriction analysis with *Sau*IIIa. CSF of patients suffering from neuroborreliosis was tested for *B. burgdorferi* DNA being present prior to and at various times subsequent to antibiotic treatment.

Methods:

Serologic analysis: All samples were analysed by flagellum ELISA Dako (Kopenhagen) and by immunoblotting with *B. burgdorferi* proteins separated on Tricine-Sodium dodecyl sulfate-polyacrylamide gel electrophoresis (Tricine-PAGE) as described by Schaegger and von Jagow. üs
Subsequently the proteins were transferred in a semi-dry condition to nitrocellulose sheets (Schleicher & Schüll, Dassel; 0.45μm) for 1.5h with a current of 0,8mA/cm^2 at room temperature.
PCR: We have developed a two-stage PCR to verify the presence of spirochaetes in the brain. 500μl of CSF was separated by centrifugation and washed. Subsequently the DNA was isolated by proteinase K and phenol/chloroform treatment. 20μl of this DNA was used as a template in a 50μl PCR preparation with the two external, flagellin specific primers, 5'-CTGCTGGCATGGGAGTTTCT-3' and 5'-TCAATTGCATACTCAG-TACT-3'. After 40 amplification cycles a second PCR run (25 cycles) was conducted with 5% of this reaction. Here two oligonucleotides, 5'-AAG-GAATTGGCAGTTCAATC-3' and 5'-ACAGCAATAGCTTCATCTTG-3', were implemented, which hybridise within the primarily amplified flagellin sequence, so that there was a subfragment of 290 bp.

Results

IgM and IgG antibodies to *B. burgdorferi* could be detected both in the CSF as well as in the serum of 19 patients with neurologic manifestations by running a a flagellin-ELISA and a tricine Western blot (WB). The sera were diluted for WB-analysis to fall in line with the IgG contents of the CSF samples (1:400 -1:500) in order to check whether CSF and serum reactivity with *B. burgdorferi* proteins varies greatly. The CSF of 14 patients reacted particularly strongly with 80 Kda, 70 Kda, 41 Kda and 38 Kda proteins. Antibodies to OspA (31Kda) could not be detected. Since the CSF in the Western blot had a more conspicious reaction pattern than the serum it seemed obvious to assume that there was a greater quantity of specific antibodies in the CSF. In order to ascertain the quantity of antibodies synthesised intrathecally, both the albumin as well as the IgG concentration in the serum and CSF were determined. The IgG/albumin (I/A) index was subsequently determined from these data according to the following formula: ((CSF IgG/serum IgG)/ (CSF albumin/ serum albumin)). The I/A index was raised in 13 patients.
The presence of spirochaetes was demonstrated in 4 of 5 seronegative patients by running a two-stage PCR approach with fla gene specific primers. To ascertain whether the amplified DNA is specific for *B. burgdorferi* and not the result of unspecific primer hybridisation, restriction analysis was conducted with *Sau*IIIa. In accordance with the restriction map of the fla gene of *B. burgdorferi* a 185bp and 105bp fragment occured.
Due to the unequivocal indications that neuroborreliosis was actually present,"Ceftriaxon" was administered intravenously (2g/daily, duration of treatment: 14 days). In the course of this therapy the PCR analysis became negative whereas *B. burgdorferi* specific antibodies still persisted.

Conclusions

- In 75% of presumed neuroborreliosis the clinical impression could be confirmed by the detection of *B. burgdorferi* specific antibodies
- Performing a two stage PCR based on the fla gene of *B. burgdorferi* spirochaetal DNA was detected in 80% of seronegative patients.
- *The nested PCR approach put us in the position to control the* effectiveness of antibiotic therapy.

166

Detection of JC Virus DNA in CSF by the Polymerase Chain Reaction

T. Weber, R. Turner, M. Burchhardt, P. Rieckmann, W. Lüer

Neurologische Klinik und Poliklinik der Universität Göttingen, Robert-Koch-Str. 40, W-3400 Göttingen

Progressive multifocal leukoencephalopathy (PML) is a rare demyelinating disorder of the central nervous system. It is caused by a human papovavirus, designated as JC (JCV) after the patient with PML whom the virus was first isolated from. With the advent of AIDS the incidence of PML has increased at least fourfold. Definite diagnosis of PML intra vitam still requires brain biopsy as the analysis of intrathecally produced virus-specific antibodies is not possible due to the lack of virus antigen. JCV-specific DNA can be detected in cerebrospinal fluid (CSF) by the polymerase chain reaction (PCR). In order to establish optimal conditions for DNA extraction and amplification from CSF a JCV-specific primer pair was designed spanning the 3' region of the large T antigen and the 3' region of the VP1 gene. Several methods were compared to release the minute amounts of viral DNA from cellfree CSF. The minimum concentration of amplifiable DNA from plasmid DNA and JC virus obtained from an infected celline was determined by PCR. These concentrations were used to spike CSF. Satisfactory amplification could be achieved with a maximum of 20% of unextracted spiked CSF in the PCR reaction buffer. Larger volumes of CSF lead to a strong inhibition of the PCR reaction. Direct salt precipitation of spiked CSF could also be used for PCR but phenol/chloroform extraction of proteinase K/ SDS treated CSF yielded much better results. The addition of salt to unextracted CSF completely abolished amplification. Adding carrier DNA or tRNA to CSF prior to extraction was generally superior to the addition of carriers before ethanol precipitation. Addition of carrier prior to extraction worked equally well for low (80 mM) and high (180 mM) salt CSF. Using a biotinylated probe after southern transfer of amplified DNA to a nylon membrane and chemiluminescence as detection system a minimum of about 100 DNA molecules per 100 μl could be demonstrated. Using a 5'-end labelled oligonucleotide as a probe in a liquid hybridization assay the lower limit of detection could further be improved. Optimal results can be obtained by adding carrier DNA to CSF prior to extraction followed by proteinase K/SDS digestion and phenol/chloroform extraction. This approach also permits the concentration of larger volumes of CSF thus further enhancing the recovery of viral DNA. Although the use of non radioactive detection systems is desirable, liquid hybridization with a radioactively labelled probe further improved sensitivity.

167

THE POLYMERASE CHAIN REACTION AS DIAGNOSTIC TOOL IN CEREBROSPINAL FLUID OF PATIENTS WITH NEUROBORRELIOSIS AND TUBERCULOUS MENINGITIS

Stephan Bamborschke*, Angelika Porr*, Brunhilde Rehse-Küpper*, Achim Kaufhold**, and Andreas Podbielski**

*Klinik für Neurologie der Universität zu Köln and **Institut für Medizinische Mikrobiologie der RWTH Aachen, FRG

Two of the most important causes of chronic meningitis are neuroborreliosis and neurotuberculosis. However, detection of *Borrelia burgdorferi* and *Mycobacterium tuberculosis* in cerebrospinal fluid (CSF) by culture is difficult, time consuming and lacks sensitivity. Thus, specific DNA amplification using the polymerase chain reaction (PCR) seems to be a promising new approach for early and reliable diagnosis in both diseases.
We performed PCR in 34 CSF samples from 13 patients with serologically proven meningopolyradiculitis Bannwarth using 3 different primer pairs (selected from DNA sequences of the Flagellin gene, the outer surface protein A gene and one conserved DNA sequence of unknown function) from *Borrelia burgdorferi*. Only in 4 patients (30%) a positive result was found. However, in one patient long-term persistence of *Borrelia burgdorferi* was detected even 2 1/2 years after penicillin treatment and normalization of the CSF cell count. After additional application of ceftriaxone PCR was negative. Thus, if initially positive, PCR may be used to evaluate the efficacy of therapeutic regimens in patients with neuroborreliosis but probably will not replace diagnostic serologic tests.
One of 3 patients with suspected tuberculous meningitis had positive PCR in CSF (primer sequence from the 65 KD heat shock protein gene of *Mycobacterium tuberculosis*). CSF culture for *Mycobacterium tuberculosis* was positive 6 weeks later. Of the remaining two PCR negative patients one was found to suffer from neurosarcoidosis and improved receiving corticosteroids, the other died of a primary leptomeningeal malignant lymphoma, which was diagnosed by autopsy. In tuberculous meningitis, PCR seems to be the most promising diagnostic approach for early and definite diagnosis which is essential for successful treatment.

168

DNA Sequence Analysis Identifies Regions Likely Responsible for Neurotropism of HIV-1

A Rolfs, I Weber, B Heidrich
Dep of Neurology (Prof. P. Marx), Klinikum Steglitz, FU Berlin, Hindenburgdamm 30, 1000 Berlin 45, Germany

In the last few years, neurological syndromes caused by the human immuno - deficiency virus type 1 (HIV-1) have increasingly become the object of intense investigations. In some cases, even a primarily intrathecal immune response can be demonstrated in the context of a fresh HIV-1 infection, while antibodies can be found in the periphery only with a latency of up to 3 months (Rolfs 1990). The detection of HIV-1 in brain tissue in endothelial and glial cells, but above all in macrophages, indicates that the virus might be responsible for numerous neuro- logical disorders found in patients with AIDS. Findings show that nerve structures, besides lymphocytes, are preferential target cells of the HIV-1 infection. Since macrophages constitute the quantitatively most important population of HIV-1-infected cells in the brain, investigations leading to findings regarding the genetic basis of the special affinity to macrophages of some HIV-1 isolates are crucial for an understanding of the so-called "neurotropism" of the virus. There are five hypervariable regions in the gene: V1 (base position) 6637-6719, V2 6744-6839, V3 7149-7233, V4 7431-7487, V5 7632-7667; moreover, the gene contains the CD4 binding site (7491-7589). Cann and co-workers (1992), in experiments using recombinant viruses, arrive at the result that the transfer of a 715bp DNA fragment from the gp120 region including the V3 loop is sufficient to alter the cell tropism of the HIV_{JR-CSF} isolate to resemble that of HIV_{NL4-J}. The mechanism by which the V3 loop might influence the cell tropism of HIV-1 could involve activation of the fusogenic potential embodied in the hydrophobic NH_2 terminus of the gp41, since the envelope fusion in HIV-1 may require a specific proteolytic activation step. Thus, the tropism would describe the ability of a cell to cleave a specific site within different V3 loops, e.g., by lysosomal proteases.
Material and methods: DNA and RNA from from peripheral blood lymphomonocytes and CSF cells has been isolated, obtained from HIV-1-positive patients displaying various stages of infection and disturbances. Using polymerase chain reaction (nested PCR) the whole HIV-1 genome from patients' isolates was succesfully amplified in approximately 25 single DNA amplification reactions using an 3'primer modified with the M13-universal sequence and a 5'primer modified with the reverse M13-universal sequence at their 5'end. The resulting PCR amplification products were subsequently sequenced without further cloning procedures (USB Corp. Sequenase™ sequencing system, ABI-dye-primer, non-radioactive sequencing procedure; for details see Rolfs 1992, pp 148-167).
Results: CSF and blood HIV-I-sequences of patients suffering from AIDS associated dementia can be distinguished by various characteristics. Special attention must here be given to the variable regions of the envelope gene region, esp. the V1 and V3 regions. In both regions, there is one respective amino-acid residue that occurs exclusively in the CSF isolates: glycine at position 147 in V1 and tyrosine at position 18 in V3. Our data demonstrate that 1. there are differences in the distribution of HIV-1 species in CSF versus blood; 2. there exist two amino acids - one in the V1 and the other in the V3 region - that might be associated closely with the determination of macrophage/monocyte tropism; 3. the genetic variation of HIV-1 in CSF cells and blood cells reaches a high level; and 4. there exist some brain-specific HIV-1 DNA sequences that were not detectable at any time in blood cells.

References
Cann AJ, Churcher MJ, Boyd M, O'Brien W, Zhao JQ, Zack J, Chen ISY (1992) The region of the envelope gene of human immunodeficiency virus type 1 responsible for determination of cell tropism. J Virol 66: 305-309

Rolfs A, Schuller I, Finckh U, Weber-Rolfs I (1992). PCR: Clinical diagnostics and research. 1992, Springer Heidelberg, New York

Rolfs A, Schumacher HC (1990). Early findings in the cerebrospinal fluid of patients with HIV-1 infection of the central nervous system. New Engl J Med 323: 418-419

169

High Number of HIV-1 Proviral Copies in Cells from Cerebrospinal Fluid

B. Wildemann, S. Munzinger, B. Storch-Hagenlocher, H. Steuler

Department of Neurology, University Hospital, Heidelberg, FRG

Human immunodeficiency virus type 1 (HIV-1) has neurotropic properties. It may directly invade the nervous system and may cause a variety of neurologic disorders. Several hypotheses are dealing with the possible role of HIV-1 in neuropathogenesis but the exact mechanism in vivo still remains unknown.

Since it is not known if neurologic dysfunction occurs in relation to the cellular infection rate in the central nervous system we determined the number of proviral copies in cells from cerebrospinal fluid (CSF) using the polymerase chain reaction (PCR). CSF from neurologically asymptomatic patients in various disease stages as well as from individuals with central nervous system infections or HIV-1 encephalopathy was included in the study.

HIV-1 DNA was found in cells from 13 of 15 CSF samples. Proviral copies were detected at a median value of 1 provirus per 300 cells with a range from 1 per 20 to 1 per 2400 cells and a mean value of 1 provirus per 500 cells. This indicates a much higher proportion of infected CSF cells than has been reported for blood mononuclear cells. However, neither the detection nor the number of HIV-1 proviral copies in CSF cells could be correlated to the disease stage or neurologic symptoms.

Poster session IV
Cerebrospinal fluid analysis
Clinical neurochemistry

170

U. Wurster, P. Lake, J. Haas:
The Specificity of CSF Oligoclonal Bands for the Diagnosis of Multiple Sclerosis

CSF-Laboratory, Neurology, Medical School Hannover, Germany

The reported occurence of so called 'false positives' in a wide range of neurological diseases threatens to discredit the reputation of the oligoclonal reaction as a diagnostic test for multiple sclerosis. Selection of patients and the kind of method chosen for separation and detection of oligoclonal bands (OB) will greatly influence the results. Criteria for oligoclonal pattern evaluation have not been properly defined and

currently one, two or three OB are taken for a positive rating. Because of the higher resolution the proved method of isoelectric focusing on 1 mm thick polyacrylamide (pH 3.5 - 9.5) gels with silverstaining is still preferred to the often recommended separation on agarose with subsequent immunoblotting. The alleged advantage of specific detection of IgG could not be confirmed for electroblotted polyacrylamide gels. While strong and intermediate OB were unequivocally identified as IgG, faint highly alkaline bands which were clearly visible in the transparent silverstained polyacrylamide gels, became blurred after electrophoretic transfer on PVDF membranes or masked by the polyclonal IgG background. Since CSF and serum are always run side by side and adjusted to equal amounts of 20 mg/l IgG , a systemic origin of OB can be easily recognized.

2200 consecutive patients were analyzed for frequency and number of OB. 1-38 bands were found in 394 (17.9 %) of all patients. A single band was observed in 46 (2.1 %) including one case of MS. Two to three bands occurred in 70 (3.2 %) patients, three of which had MS and three had isolated optic neuritis.Thus, only four (2.5 %) of the 161 cases with MS (a further three were negative) did not reach the chosen limit of four bands, yet for optic neuritis already three (14.3 %) of the 21 patients with OB stayed below the cut-off value. The number of OB in MS correlated with the amount of local IgG synthesis (IgG Index, r = 0.75). The importance of an appropriate decision limit can be recognized from the 10 cases of brain infarct with OB where only two exhibited more than four bands, or the seven cases of vertigo with OB where none surpassed the cut-off, but six had a single band. Since the expression of OB in the CSF indicates an ongoing immune response in the CNS , quite obviously their presence cannot be entirely specific for MS. After elimination of infectious CNS diseases and by the application of the conservative criterion of at least four unique CSF bands, the specificity for MS reaches 97.4 % while the sensitivity is 96 %. Lowering the cut-off to one band, only marginally improves sensitivity to 98.2 %, but specificity decreases to 93 %. If autoimmune disorders like Sharp syndrome, SLE, Sjögren syndrome ,inflammatory (sarcoidosis, Tolosa-Hunt syndrome) and lymphoproliferative diseases are also subtracted, the proportion of so-called 'false positives' will drop to 1.9 %. The number of OB is usually low in this group and quantitative elevation of IgG synthesis is rarely observed. Nevertheless among the majority of cases an intrathecal immune reaction can be imagined. An anamnestic reaction may have remained after previous (subclinical) involvement of the CNS in systemic infectious diseases. Basal ganglia diseases or epilepsy associated with weak OB may represent monosymptomatic MS, especially when a single lesion in the appropriate anatomic region can be demonstrated in brain magnetic resonance imaging. Another mechanism might be the unspecific and time-limited stimulation of IgG synthesis elicited by mitogenic factors, set free in the course of tissue destruction i.e. in brain infarcts, an interpretation strengthened by the observation of two to three OB in 2/10 cases with brain contusion. Finally, mounting of an immune reaction against tumor or cross-reactive antigens appears possible in primary and secondary brain tumors as well as in paraneoplastic diseases.

171

SPECIFIC AND UNSPECIFIC DETECTION OF OLIGOCLONAL BANDS IN CEREBROSPINAL FLUID (CSF) FROM PATIENTS WITH INFLAMMATORY DISEASES OF CENTRAL NERVOUS SYSTEM (CNS) UTILIZING PHASTSYSTEM (PHARMACIA-LKB)

Rolf HACKLER and Tilmann O. KLEINE

Med. Zentrum für Nervenheilkunde, Neurologische Klinik (Funktionsbereich Neurochemie) der Universität, Rudolf Bultmannstr. 8, D-W-3550 Marburg/Lahn, Germany

<u>Introduction</u>: Examination of CSF for the occurrence of oligoclonal bands (OB) (in comparison to serum) is a well established laboratory test in the diagnosis of inflammatory diseases of CNS. Isoelectric focusing (IEF) in polyacrylamide gels and silver staining are frequently used to detect OB because of high resolution and sensitivity. Conventional IEF methods utilizing unconcentrated CSF are time consuming and difficult to reproduce. Therefore we developed a reproducible routine method, easy and quick to perform, for the specific and semi-automated detection of OB in small amounts of unconcentrated CSF (1-5). The influence of different precipitation techniques (unspecific and specific) to detect OB were investigated.

<u>Methods</u>: Separation of proteins was done by (IEF) in PhastSystemTM using ready made polyacrylamide gels PhastGelTM IEF 3-9. To increase the resolution of bands and to expand the pH gradient in the alkaline region gels were modified as described (1, 2, 4). To increase the sensitivity and number of samples per gel a special applicator with 10 sample slots (each 4 μl) was used. Automated silver staining was performed in PhastSystemTM as described (4) after unspecific precipitation of proteins by trichloroacetic acid or after specific precipitation by monospecific antisera (AS) against human IgG (γ-chain), Ig light chains of λ or $\varkappa$ type (free and bound) and removing of unprecipitated material by washing.

<u>Results and discussion:</u> Applying these modifications of PhastSystemTM to native CSF samples the resolution of bands was better than that in conventional gels or unmodified PhastGelTM. Optimum results were obtained in 4 μl sample with an IgG content of 20 mg/l using unspecific silver staining, resp. 8 mg/l applying specific immunofixation followed by silver staining. Detection limit of one band was 600 pg IgG with the former resp. 150 pg IgG with the latter method. In some cases additional bands were only detectable using immunofixation. Additional bands after silver staining (not obtained with immunofixation) made the detection less specific yielding no definite results. Thus immunofixation gives a clearly positive result even in cases with one additional specific band in contrast to unspecific band detection with silver staining where different numbers of additional bands are used as criterion for OB. In summary IEF with immunofixation in modified PhastSystemTM offers an optimum method for the specific detection of OB in native human CSF.

References:
1. Hackler R, Kleine TO (1987) Darstellung oligokonaler Banden in nativen unkonzentrierten Liquorproben durch Modifikation des PhastSystemTM (Pharmacia). Lab med 11: 176
2. Hackler R, Kleine TO (1988) Flattening and/or expanding of pH gradients in isoelectric focusing gels exemplified with PhastSystem. Electrophoresis 9: 262-267
3. Hackler R, Kleine TO, Schlenska GK (1989) Automated isoelectric focusing (IEF) and immuno-detection of oligoclonal bands in unconcentrated CSF: Comparison with agarose gel electrophoresis. J Clin Chem Clin Biochem 27: 909-910
4. Hackler R, Kleine TO (1991) Modifikation des PhastSystemTM zum automatisierten Nachweis oligoklonaler Banden im nativen Liquor cerebrospinalis durch IEF mit Immundetektion. Lab med 15: 185-192
5. Hackler, R., Kleine, T.O. (1992) Evaluation of immunoreactivity of human central nervous system: Automated determination of oligoclonal IgG bands versus calculation of intrathecal IgG production. In: Wegmann RJ, Wegmann MA (eds) Recent advances in cellular and molecular biology, vol 3, Peeters Press, Leuven (in press)

172

Intrathecal synthesis of immunoglobulins and virus-specific antibodies in inflammatory neurologic diseases.

M. Näher-Noé, J. Klingelhöfer, S. Freytag, B. Conrad

Department of Neurology, Technical University of Munich, Möhlstraße 28, W-8000 München 80

The determination of intrathecal IgG-synthesis and oligoclonal bands in CSF is an indicator of inflammatory neurologic disease but does not allow a differentiation between different inflammatory diseases. We therefore examined, whether the determination of intrathecal synthesis of IgA and IgM, as well as virus-specific antibodies, is helpful in the differentiation between inflammatory diseases.

We analysed 168 unselected paired CSF and serum samples of patients with clinically definite (45) and probable multiple sclerosis (22), isolated optic neuritis (5), acute (16) and chronic neuroborreliosis (4), other inflammatory (40) and noninflammatory neurologic diseases (36). In addition to routine CSF analysis including cytology, determination of glucose, total protein, albumin, IgG and oligoclonal immunoglobulins, we measured IgA and IgM in serum and CSF by enzyme immunoassay. We also determined antibodies for measles, rubella and varicella zoster by enzyme immunoassay in CSF and serum. Intrathecal synthesis of a specific virus antibody was assumed if the specific CSF/serum ratio was higher than 2.5.

For definite and probable multiple sclerosis we found pleocytosis in 26%, oligoclonal immunoglobulins in 98% and intrathecal synthesis of IgG in 81%, IgA in 15% and IgM in 15% of the patients. For acute and chronic neuroborreliosis pleocytosis was found in 75%, increased total protein and albumin in 65%, oligoclonal immunoglobulin in 80%, intrathecal synthesis of IgG in 45%, IgA in 25% and IgM in 55% of the patients. Patients with noninflammatory neurologic diseases had normal CSF except for an increase of total protein and albumin in patients with spinal stenosis. We found intrathecal synthesis of at least one of the three virus antibodies in definite multiple sclerosis in 87%, probable multiple sclerosis in 55% and isolated optic neuritis in 40% of the patients. Regarding neuroborreliosis, virus antibodies were found in all 4 patients with chronic neuroborreliosis, but in none of those with acute neuroborreliosis. In the group with other inflammatory neurologic diseases only 1 patient (herpes encephalitis) showed antibodies to varicella zoster; all other patients with inflammatory diseases and all those with noninflammtory diseases were negative for intrathecal virus antibody synthesis.

Intrathecal synthesis of IgM seems to be common in neuroborreliosis, in contrast to multiple sclerosis. Intrathecal synthesis of virus-specific antibodies in absence of a viral infection is typical for multiple sclerosis and chronic neuroborreliosis, in sharp contrast to acute neuroborreliosis and other inflammatory diseases. It might be speculated, that the immunological reaction in chronic neuroborreliosis is different from that in acute neuroborreliosis and rather resembles part of the immunological phenomena in multiple sclerosis. Certainly, the determination of IgA, IgM and virus-specific antibodies is important in the differential diagnosis of inflammatory diseases of the CNS.

173

Observation of T-lymphocyte receptors and cytokines in the peripheral blood (PB) of patients with relapse remitting multiple sclerosis (RRMS)

S. Schimrigk [1,2], R. Lange [1,2], H.W. Kölmel [2]

1) Department of Neurology, Universitätsklinikum Rudolf Virchow, Freie Universität - Berlin, Germany
2) Department of Neurology, Charité, Humboldt University, Berlin, Germany

Introduction:
Peripheral blood lymphocyte (PBL) activation plays an important role in the immunopathogenesis of multiple sclerosis (MS). Cytokines such as interleukin 1ß (IL-1ß), interleukin 2 (IL-2) with its corresponding receptor (CD25) and HLA-DR are mediators in the immunoregulation of T-helper lymphocytes. IL-1ß secreted by macrophages and IL-2 secreted by T-helper lymphocytes stimulate the expression of the CD25 receptor. According to the theory of peripheral T-lymphocyte activation, lymphocytes migrate into the brain where they are involved in the demyelination process (1, 2). In this study, we looked for activated CD25 + T-lymphocytes and cytokines in the PB of untreated patients with RRMS. The correlations between the laboratory findings and the clinical status were considered.

Methods:
Over the course of 14 days, every second day, blood and sera were collected from 5 patients with clinical and laboratory defined RRMS who are undergoing a relapse state. Five patients with inflammatory diseases of the nervous system and 5 healthy subjects served as control groups. The levels of the IL-1ß and IL-2 concentrations were evaluated by ELISA technique (Quantikine, R&D Systems, Mineapolis). T-lymphocyte receptor expression was measured by using monoclonal antibodies directed to CD4, CD8, CD25 and HLA-DR (all from DAKO, Kopenhagen, Denmark). The samples were analysed using double staining technique (Facscan, Becton Dickinson). The clinical status of analysed patients was classified by EDSS (Kurtzke, 1983).

Results:
The results showed no detectable levels of IL-1ß and IL-2 in tested sera. There was no evidence for peripheral T-cell activation studying MS patients. Also the course of receptor fluctuation as the percentage of CD25 + T-cells did not prove any correlation with the clinical findings, duration of the disease and the EDSS. The effectiveness of monitoring the levels of CD25 receptor expression as well as the amount of IL-1ß and IL-2 concentrations in PB in patients with RRMS did not reveal positive or negative correlation.

Discussion:
A relapse in MS caused by activated PBLs is not detectable by measuring elevated CD25 receptor expression or cytokine concentrations. There are two possible explanations for the lack of elevated CD25 receptor levels in the PB of patients with RRMS: (i) migration of activated T-lymphocytes into lymphatic tissue or (ii) crossing the blood-brain-barrier and invading into the brain tissue. Our data implicate that recently discussed reactivation of PBL´s in patients with RRMS is questionable.

References:
1. Hafler DA and Weiner HL (1989) MS: A CNS and systemic autoimmune disease. Immunology today 10 (3): 104.
2. Wucherpfennig KW, Weiner HL, Hafler DA (1991) T-cell recognition of myelin basic protein. Immunology today 12 (8): 277-282.

174

Prognostic Factors for the Effect of Corticoid-Therapy in Multiple Sclerosis (MS)

Kwiet K.-D., Rüttinger H., Schimrigk K.
University of Saarland, Department of Neurology
D-6650 Homburg/Saar

The significance of certain clinical features for the long-term-prognosis of multiple sclerosis (MS) is well established; these include the clinical course and clinical type, age of onset, relapse frequency and the patient's sex. In an open prospective clinical trial we tried to find the decisive factors for the short-term-effect of a corticoid-therapy in MS-patients with either acute relapse or chronic detioration of their disease.

152 patients with LSDMS (laboratory-supported definite multiple sclerosis) were randomly assigned to one of two therapeutic regimen: either intravenous methylprednisolone (MP) (starting with 100 mgs) or triamcinolonacetonide (TA) 40 mg, given intrathecally three times, once a week. Mean age of the patients was 31 ys, mean disease duration 6 ys, the sex ratio was 1 : 1,7 ($\male$: $\female$). Disability profile was assesed with EDSS and FS (Kurtzke) and Ambulation-Index (Hauser) at the beginning of therapy and three weeks later; CSF was taken before therapy and with each further lumbar puncture in the TA patients.

The results of the study show that many other factors have more importance for the effect of corticoid-therapy than the choice of the substance itself and the way of application. A good outcome ($0,85 \leq \Delta EDSS < 1,15$) was found in patients with the following characteristics: disease duration ≤ 1 y, relapsing-remitting course, CSF pleocytosis, early begin of the therapy in relation to onset of the symptoms, age ≤ 25 ys, female sex and EDSS ≤ 4. Unsatisfactory results ($\Delta EDSS \leq 0,5$) were obtained in chronic-progressive courses of the disease, disease duration > 5 ys, male sex, EDSS > 4 and late begin of the therapy. The age of onset had only a poor influence on the effect of therapy compared to disease duration. Acute sensory symptoms responded better to treatment than motor or even cerebellar symptoms. What however the two therapeutic regimen are concerned, they were equal regarding all parameters mentioned above. The only difference was found in relation to the amount of locally produced IgG (IgG_{loc}): the effect under intrathecally given TA was the better the more IgG_{loc} was measured. In contrast, the effect of intravenous MP was not influenced by the amount of IgG_{loc}.

Since clinical features exert such a great influence on therapeutic effects, they have always to be considered when testing the effect of a certain substance.

175

Intrathecal Treatment with Triamcinolon-Acetonide Reduces Central Nervous System IgG Synthesis in Patients with Chronic Progressive Multiple Sclerosis

L. Schöls,

D. Pöhlau, J. Wagener, T. Postert, H. Przuntek
Neurologic clinic, St. Josef Hospital, Ruhr-University Bochum, Germany

Chronic progressive type of multiple sclerosis has an especially pure prognosis and immunsuppressive agents mostly fail to be therapeutically effective.

We studied the effect of intrathecal steroid treatment on immunological parameters in 20 patients with multiple sclerosis of chronic progressive type. Triamcinolon-acetonide (TCA) was given intrathecally after lumbar puncture. Every patient received injections of 40 mg TCA soluted in 10 ml NaCl 0.9% twice a week for 3 weeks. CSF was analysed for white cell count, total protein, albumin, IgG, IgM and IgA fraction at the first and last injection. Autochthone IgG production was calculated using the formula of Reiber [1].

Cell count in CSF tends to increase, probably because of iatrogenic stimulation, but increase did not reach statistical significance. Total protein content of CSF and plasma did not change. Albumin content of CSF decreased while plasma albumin kept stable resulting in a signifantly improved CSF/serum ratio for albumin. For IgG CSF/serum ratio decreased significantly, too. No patient had signs of blood-brain barrier dysfunction alowing calculation of intrathecal IgG production according to the formula of Reiber [1]: The autochthone IgG production was reduced significantly.

TCA level in CSF taken before the sixth TCA injection reached 400 fold the level of plasma TCA taken at the same time.

These results are interpreted as strong hints of immunological efficiency of intrathecal steroid therapy in chronic progressive multiple sclerosis.

Literature:
1. Reiber H (1980) The discrimination between different blood-CSF barrier dysfunctions and inflammatory reactions of the CNS by a recent evaluation graph for the protein profile of CSF. J Neurol 224: 89

176

Multiple Sclerosis: Reaction of IgG and IgM after intrathecally given Triamcinolon

M. Wachinger, G. Holzer, K. Schimrigk
Universitätsnervenklinik, Klinische Neurochemie 6650 Homburg/Saar

Introduction: The medication of MS patients with glucocorticoids as immunosuppressive agents is believed to be a causal therapy. To avoid the unwanted systemic hormonal effects we give the hardly soluble triamcinolone acetonide as lumbal deposit. The therapeutical effect on the production of intrathecal IgG, IgM and on other immunological parameters was examinated.

Methods: A group of 103 patients (71 females, mean age was 38 years) with definitely diagnosed MS and supposed recent relapse were studied retrospectively. They had an intrathecal therapy with 40 mg Volon^{R}A (Squibb-Heyden), 3times with one week intervals. Three CSF were taken with weekly intervals: before therapy, then immediately before the second and before the last Volon medication. Albumin, IgG and C 4 (in serum only) were measured with the Behring nephelometer. IgM concentrations were determined with a home made ELISA in normal sandwich technique and peroxydase as marker enzyme. To quantitate the intrathecally synthesised immunoglobulins we used the IgG-index (Delpech-Lichtblau, normally lower than 0.6) and the IgM index (normally lower than 0.08).

Results and discussion: Increased IgG index was found in 86% and increased IgM index in 61% of the untreated patients. The mean values of the indices were 1,21 (minimal value 0.01 and maximal 3.2) and 0.2 (minimal 0.01, maximal 3.2) respectively. One week after the first Volon application the mean IgG index had slightly fallen (9%) which was a significant effect (Wilcoxon test, p = 0.025). The great majority of the patients (59%) had a diminished IgG synthesis after this week, in 41% of the patients the index had risen. The course of the local IgM synthesis was not in parallel with the IgG trend. We could find a slight increase of the mean IgM index after the first week (7%, not significant). Two equal groups with falling (43% of patients) or increasing tendency (45%) could be listed.
A risen immunoglobulin production was the effect of the second Volon treatment. This was true in 50% of the patients in regard to the IgG, whereas 46% had a decreased IgG synthesis. The overall effect of the two Volon administrations was a 2.4% decrease in the IgG index (significance , p = 0.062). The mean IgM index had further increased after the second Volon instillation (12% in total, significant with p = 0.059).
Serum IgG was the only parameter which decreased continuously following the Volon therapy. After 2 weeks the IgG mean concentration had fallen with a highly significant 8.9 % effect. The concentration of complement (C 4) in serum did not show correlation with the tendency of the immunoglobulins in serum or in CSF. The established weak effect of the intrathecal therapy on immunity parameters could be declared by the very local application of the triamcinolone and the delayed release from the lumbal deposit. The slight but significant depression of serum IgG at least is remarkable, the relation of this small immunosuppressive effect with clinical improvement is not yet clear.

177

ANALYSIS AND ASSESSMENT OF A THREE ARMED STUDY ON PASSIVE IMMUNOTHERAPY IN MULTIPLE SCLEROSIS

H. Meyer-Rienecker, E. Schmitt, E. Behm, M. Palm, B. Hitzschke, K. Lakner, G. Kundt
Dept. of Neurology and Dept. of Internal Medicine, University of Rostock

In contrast to the non-specific immunosuppression and the active immunostimulation, the passive immunotherapy, such as the therapeutic plasma exchange (TPE) and the immunoadsorption (IA) aims at the removal of serum factors (e.g. antibodies, pathogenic autoantigens, interleukins, complement and other factors) to influence the disturbances of immunoregulation in MS.

Altogether 30 **patients** with clinically definite MS (1) were treated. Randomization was performed by a computerized blocked program concerning several parameters (sex, age, onset of disease), esp. the activity, i.e. acute exacerbation or chronic progressive course.
The study concerns **three groups**:
1. Group P: Corticosteroids; Prednisolone 60 mg/d iv./7d, reduction (5 mg)/4 weeks (= BT, basic therapy).
2. Group TPE: Therapeutic plasma exchange; 4 TPE/8 d, 50 ml/kg body weight, 5 % Human Albumin (Biotest) + BT.
3. Group IA: Immunoadsorption; 4 IA/8 d, Immusorba PH-350 (IM-PH) columns, Plasmaflo HI 05 (ASAHI Med. Co., Tokyo), 50 ml/kg body weight + BT.

Measurements of impairments were performed using EDSS and FS (Kurtzke). A value of effectivity (VE) was calculated, i.e. the differences between the FS scores before and after therapy: positive values indicate improvement, negative ones progression.

The **follow up** of EDSS and FS in cases of attacks of MS showed a marked improvement for at least 3 months in the TPE and IA group. In patients of chronic-progressive course recovery was rare and transitory. Generally after 52 weeks no improvement could be observed: this especially concerns in the relapsing-remitting form the IA group, in the chronic progressive course the P group.

VE weeks	Acute exacerbation			Chronic progressive course		
	P	TPE	IA	P	TPE	IA
2	0.27	0.65	0.72	0.28	0.10	0.37
12	0.17	0.80	1.06	-0.06	0.10	0.33
52	0.04	0.40	-0.13	-0.37	0.05	0.03

The **results** were still more distinct applying the mean VE (see Table). In (a.) case of acute exacerbation they were higher in group TPE than in group P, and considerably higher in group IA; but this held true only for a limited period, i.e. some months: one year after beginning of procedures, lower values were noticed in all three groups, even to negative values in the group IA. In (b.) chronic progressive forms of disease the progression could not be influenced.
In regard to the rare investigations of the **mechanisms** of TPE and IA, the discovery of the behaviour of the plasma IgG, IgM, IgA, fibrinogen and complement factors (Clq, Cl-INH, C4, C3, C9), the total hemolytic activities (THC) - classic (CH 50) and alternative pathway (3) was determined. The levels of above mentioned proteins in TPE group were rapidly decreased, up to 75 %, in case of IA slightly diminished, by about 20 %. The hemolytic capacities of the complement system showed a decrease in both treatment procedures up to 75 %.

Summarizing could be stated: (1.) In the acute phases of MS the TPE and IA treatments are more effective than corticosteroids alone. (2.) The activity of MS can be influenced for only a limited period of time, but not at all so the dynamics and course of the disease. (3.) Our additional analyses revealed that the therapeutic effect of TPE and IA may be achieved by the reduction of complement activity. (4.) It is hardly possible to influence the chronic progressive course of MS.

1. Hitzschke B, Meyer-Rienecker HJ, Buddenhagen F, Richter M (1988) Psychiat Neurol med Psychol 40: 598-608
2. Meyer-Rienecker H (1991) Neurologija 40 Suppl 1: 15-22
3. Palm M, Behm E, Schmitt E, Buddenhagen F, Hitzschke B, Kracht M, Kundt G, Meyer-Rienecker H, Klinkmann H (1991) *Biomat Artif Cells Immob Biotech* 19: 283-296

178

ACTIVATION MARKERS ON FETAL-TYPE LYMPHOCYTES IN CEREBROSPINAL FLUID OF PATIENTS WITH NEUROIMMUNOLOGICAL DISEASES

E.Mix*[&], U.Fiszer*, T.Olsson*, S.Fredrikson*, V.Kostulas*, H.Meyer-Rienecker[&], H.Link*
* Dept. of Neurology, Karolinska Institute, Huddinge University Hospital, Stockholm, Sweden
[&] Dept. of Neurology, Hospital for Nervous Diseases, University of Rostock, Germany

Fetal-type lymphocytes are defined as $CD5^+$ B cells and $\gamma\delta^+$ T cells [1]. They have been found to be increased in cerebrospinal fluid of patients with multiple sclerosis (MS) and other inflammatory neurological diseases (OIND) compared to noninflammatory controls (CO) [1, 2]. In this study we investigated by three-color flow cytometry $CD5^+$ B cells and $\gamma\delta^+$ T cells for their expression of activation markers CD25, IL-2 receptor p75 (IL2-Rß), adhesion molecules CD11a, CD18, CD44 and CD54, and the 'epithelial' δTCS1 subtype of $\gamma\delta^+$ T cells in CSF and blood of patients with MS (N=15), OIND (N=17) and CO (N=13).
In CSF CD25 and CD54 were expressed on $\gamma\delta^+$ T cells in 5/11, resp. 9/11, of MS patients, in 9/16, resp. 9/16, of OIND patients, and 2/9, resp. 2/5, of CO patients. In blood the frequency of $CD25^+$ and $CD54^+$ $\gamma\delta^+$ T cells was 1/15 and 7/13 in MS, 6/17 and 6/17 in OIND, and 3/11 and 2/11 in CO.
In CSF and blood of patients with MS and OIND $CD5^+$ B cells expressed higher levels of CD25 than conventional $CD5^-$ B cells (Table 1).

Table 1. CD25 expression on $CD5^+$ B cells in CSF and blood of patients with inflammatory diseases of the nervous system[a]

	MS		OIND	
	CSF	blood	CSF	blood
$CD5^+$ B cells	30.0 + 9.1	19.5 + 8.2	22.5 + 9.7	18.5 + 8.9
$CD5^-$ B cells	16.2 + 4.9	10.6 + 5.1	13.8 + 6.9	9.7 + 5.2

[a]Values represent mean SD of the percentages of CD25 expressing cells within the $CD5^+$ and $CD5^-$ B cell subpopulations.

IL2-Rß was only expressed on $CD5^+$ B cells, i.e. on 6.4%, resp. 5.0%, in CSF and on 2.8%, resp. 2.4%, in blood in MS, resp. OIND.

CD11a and CD18 expression as measured by relative fluorescence intensity was higher on $\gamma\delta^+$ than on $\gamma\delta^-$ T cells in blood of all patients. In CSF CD11a and CD18 expression was not significantly different between $\gamma\delta^+$ and $\gamma\delta^-$ T cells, but CD18 expression was higher on $\gamma\delta^+$ than on $\gamma\delta^-$ T cells in MS. Between patient groups the only significant difference was higher CD11a expression on CSF $\gamma\delta^-$ T cells in MS compared to OIND. CD44 was more expressed on $\gamma\delta^+$ than on $\gamma\delta^-$ T cells in CSF of MS patients, and $\gamma\delta^+$ blood T cells expressed more CD44 in MS than in CO. In blood there was no difference in CD44 expression between $\gamma\delta^+$ and $\gamma\delta^-$ T cells. Only a minority of $\gamma\delta^+$ T cells in CSF and blood was δTCS1$^+$ with the lowest values (mean 25%) in MS. This finding is in accordance with low occurrence of δTCS1$^+$ T cells in MS brain tissue [3], but it contrasts with increased blood and synovial δTCS1$^+$ T cell levels in rheumatoid arthritis [4]. We conclude that $CD5^+$ B cells are selectively activated in inflammatory neurological diseases, whereas fetal-type $\gamma\delta^+$ T cells are only partially activated with sequestration to the CSF compartment. They seem to support the chronicity of inflammatory processes in the central nervous system. The majority of $\gamma\delta^+$ T cells does not belong to the 'epithelial' δTCS1 subtype, which may rather play a role in nondemyelinating inflammation [4]. Since in MS $\gamma\delta^+$ T cells seem neither to be of 'blood-borne' Vδ2 subtype [5], selective expansion of a so far undefined subtype is suggestive.
This work was supported by the Swedish Association of Neurological Disabled, Stockholm, and the Hertie Foundation, Frankfurt.

1. Correale J, Mix E, Olsson T, Kostulas V, Fredrikson S, Höjeberg B, Link H (1991) J Neuroimmunol 32:123-132
2. Mix E, Correale J, Olsson T, Kostulas V, Fredrikson S, Höjeberg B, Link H (1991) Lab Med 15: 79-81
3. Selmay K, Brosnan CF, Raine CS (1991) Proc Natl Acad Sci USA 88: 6452-6456
4. Keystone EC, Rittershaus C, Wood N, Snow KM, Flatow J, Purvis JC, Poplonski L, Kung PC (1991) Clin Exp Immunol 84: 78-82
5. De Libero G, Uematsu Y, Kappos L (1992) Neurology 42 (Suppl. 3): 246

179

New Tumor Markers in CSF: c-erbB-2/neu Oncoprotein and mutant p53 Suppressor Gene Product

M. Schabet, H. Wiethölter, E. Dubois, J. Dichgans

Neurologische Universitätsklinik, Hoppe-Seyler-Strasse 3, W-7400 Tübingen, Federal Republic of Germany

The cellular oncogen erbB-2/neu codes for a membrane-bound protein (Erb-2/Neu) related to the epidermal growth factor receptor. Its natural ligand is hitherto unknown. Erb-2/Neu is overexpressed and shedded into circulation mainly in breast and ovarian carcinomas but also in other carcinomas and malignant tumors [1, 2]. The p53 suppressor gene physiologically controls cell division. It has been found to be mutated in the majority of human cancers. Compared with its physiological counterpart the mutant dys- or non-functioning protein (mP53) has a considerably increased half-life time and therefore accumulates within tumor cells. It is released upon cell death [3]. The potential role of mP53 and ErbB-2/Neu as tumor markers in body fluids has not been elucidated so far. Using commercially available ELISAs we therefore measured both proteins in the CSF of non-tumorous control patients and of patients with cytologically diagnosed neoplastic meningitis (NM).

ErbB-2/Neu measured 45 ± 19 human Neu units (HNU)/ml in 14 controls (3 normal, 1 subarachnoid hemorrhage, 3 multiple sclerosis, 7 bacterial meningitis), and 866 ± 2406 HNU/ml in 34 cases of NM. ErbB-2/Neu was significantly elevated above the mean value plus three standard deviations of controls in 19 of the 34 patients with NM (7/11 breast cancer, 6/8 lung cancer, 2/4 non-Hodgkin lymphoma, 1/4 melanoma, 3/7 other malignancies). In 21 cases of NM, ErbB-2 and albumin were measured both in CSF and in serum. Considering the CSF/serum concentration quotients of both proteins the same individual specimens as pointed out above showed significantly elevated or normal values when compared with the controls except for 3 cases (2 cases turned pathological, 1 normal). Elevated ErbB-2/Neu did not correlate with prognosis.

The non-tumorous control CSF specimens were negative for mP53. It measured 0.46 ± 0.26 ng/ml, however, in 6 of 10 cases of NM diagnosed in 1990 and 1991 (1/2 breast cancer, 1/3 lung cancer, 1/1 cervical cancer, 0/1 melanoma, 1/1 myelosarcoma, 1/1 medul-loblastoma). Three corresponding serum samples also showed mP53 (breast cancer, lung cancer, myelosarcoma). In contrast to Erb-2/Neu no mP53 was detected in 21 older CSF specimens which had repeatedly been thawn and refrozen.

We estimate that combined measurement of mP53 and c-ErbB-2/Neu in fresh CSF yields relevant pathological findings in about 70% of patients with NM. Therefore, mP53 and ErbB-2/Neu are promising CSF tumor markers and should be further evaluated.

1. Slamon DJ, Gogolphin W, Jones LA, Holt J, Wong SG, Keith DR, Levin W, Stuart SG, Udove J, Ullrich A, Press MF (1989) Studies of the HER-2/neu proto-oncogene in human breast and ovarian cancer. Science 244:707-712

2. Zabrecky JR, Lam T, McKenzie SJ, Carney W (1991) The extracellular domain of p185/neu is released from the surface of human breast carcinoma cells, SK-BR-3. J Biol Chem 266:1716-1720

3. Levine AJ, Momand JM, Finlay CA (1991) The p53 tumour suppressor gene. Nature 351:453-456

180

SENSITIVE DETERMINATION OF CEA-SYNTHESIS IN CEREBROSPINAL FLUID (CSF) COMPARED WITH CSF CYTOLOGY IN DETECTION OF CARCINOMA INFILTRATION OF CENTRAL NERVOUS SYSTEM (CNS)

Wick M.[1], Huber M.[1], Einhäupl K.[2], Jehn U.[3], Fateh-Moghadam A.[1]

[1] Institute for Clinical Chemistry, [2] Department of Neurology, [3] III Medical Department of Klinikum Großhadern, University of Munich, Marchioninistr. 15, D-8000 MÜNCHEN 70, F.R.G.

CNS carcinoma involvement requires local chemotherapy and/or irradiation depending on the type of infiltration. However, sensitivity of CSF cytology (1) and specificity of imaging methods are not sufficient to detect meningeal and cerebral carcinoma metastases in all cases. All 208 patients examined over a 3-year-period for presumed CNS infiltration by solid tumours had simultaneous spinal and venipunctures to compare the diagnostic value of high-sensitivity determinations of CEA-Synthesis in CNS with WRIGHT-stained cytospin preparations of CSF cells. Of these patients, 24 had meningeal carcinomatosis, 17 cerebral carcinoma metastases without leptomeningeal infiltration, 10 extradural carcinoma metastases, 9 CNS involvement of mesenchymal tumours, 23 primary brain tumours. In contrast to that, in 47 patients with tumours of various origin and histology a CNS involvement could be definitely excluded, further 53 had benign or functional CNS diseases and in 25 CNS tumour involvement remained ambiguous.

CEA in CSF and serum was determined by a modified, high-sensitive (detection limit 0,02 ng/ml, within run CV: 10,6% at 0,086 ng/ml) monoclonal sandwich-type ELISA (Enzygnost CEA micro, Behringwerke Marburg, F.R.G.) based on microtitration plates. Modifications to enhance sensitivity were as follows: 2 step- instead of one-step-assay, increased period of sample incubation (20 h), increased amount of sample. CEA-synthesis in CNS was considered proven, if the CEA CSF/serum ratio surmounted the albumin CSF/serum ratio as a barrier indicator, determined by immunonephelometry, according to Reiber's and Felgenhauer's principles (2).

For detection of meningeal carcinomatosis, at 100% specificity level, sensitivity was found at 75% for CEA-synthesis, 79% for cytology and 96% for cytology and CEA combined. This means a positive predictive value (PV) of 1,0 in all cases compared to a negative PV of 0,96 for both CEA and cytology and of 0,99 for CEA and cytology combined. Carcinoma metastases without meningeal exfoliation were detectable only by CEA-synthesis with a sensitivity of 65% at 100% specificity, while results of imaging methods were positive in 24%, ambiguous in 47% or negative in 29%. This means a positive PV of 1,0 compared to a negative PV of 0,87 for cytology and 0,96 for CEA alone and in combination with cytology. No correlation between tumour cell count and locally produced CEA fraction was found, emphasizing the diagnostic independence of these parameters. Tumour infiltration of non-epithelial origin did not cause a local CEA-production in any case; whereas in 16% a meningeal tumour cell exfoliation was found.

We conclude, that sensitive detection of CEA-synthesis in CSF can enhance the recognition of meningeal carcinomatosis towards very high sensitivity at 100 % specificity compared to cytology alone. Furthermore, CEA-Synthesis may contribute to a more specific detection of purely intracerebral carcinoma metastases in cases with ambiguous results of imaging methods. However, this requires a barrier dependent evaluation of results and a high-sensitive determination of CEA not provided by unmodified commercial immunoassays. The method evaluated in this study enabled a similar diagnostic sensitivity, but a higher practicability for routine purposes than the first method (2) meeting the requirements mentioned above. The lack of correlation between tumour cell load and CEA production is probably due to differences in CEA synthesis in individual tumours and in location-dependent pathways of CSF resorption.

We thank Friedrich-Baur-Foundation, Munich, and Dr. Pfleiderer, Behringwerke, Marburg, F.R.G., for their support.

1) Oehmichen M., 1976 Cerebrospinal fluid cytology. An introduction and atlas Georg Thieme Publishers Stuttgart

2) Reiber H., Jacobi C., Felgenhauer K. (1986) Sensitive quantitation of carcinoembryonic antigen and its barrier-dependent differentiation. Clin. Chim. Acta 156: 259-270

181

COMPARISON OF HETTICH CENTRIFUGATION AND SAYK SEDIMENTATION FOR EXAMINATION OF CEREBROSPINAL FLUID CELLS

R.Lehmitz, H.Meyer-Rienecker
Department of Neurology, Hospital for Nervous
Diseases, University of Rostock

The most commonly used techniques for preparation of cerebrospinal fluid (CSF) cells are centrifugation and sedimentation. Cell recovery and results of cell differentiation depend essentially on the technique used for cell enrichment [1]. This has consequences for diagnostic conclusions drawn from results of cytological examination. Therefore, we compared the cell enrichment techniques by Hettich cytocentrifuge and by conventional sedimentation chamber.

The two-step technique (precentrifugation of CSF samples for cell concentration and subsequent centrifugation by Hettich cytocentrifuge) yields cell preparations, which are of good quality and easy to differentiate with a recovery rate of about 50% (range 30-70%). High recovery requires careful and reproducible handling of samples during cell resuspension and removal of cell-free CSF. Satisfying quality of cells is only achieved, if protein is added to the cell suspension prior to cytocentrifugation, e.g. bovine serum albumin solution of final concentration 40 g/l. If cell-free CSF is removed remaining a defined quantity of fluid and resuspension is performed without addition of protein, an unsatisfactory cell quality with numerous cell ghosts is resulting, especially in cases of low cell count and low protein content. The method allows to provide several cell preparations for cytological and immunocytochemical stainings even at cell counts <5 Mpt/l. The results of cell differentiation reflect the _in vivo_ conditions with approximately 85% lymphocytes and approximately 15% monocytes in "normal" CSF. In cell-rich preparations yielded by cytocentrifuge it is more probable to detect cells of diagnostic relevance, which are present at low quantity, e.g. plasma cells and "activated" B cells in chronic inflammatory diseases of the nervous system. Likewise detection of tumor cells is facilitated. However, large and relatively labil cells, like "erythrophages", can be destroyed by the procedure of cytocentrifugation and may lead to a false negative assertion of phagocytosis of erythrocytes in cases of hemorrhage into the cerebrospinal space.

Results of preparations by sedimentation according to the standard method of SAYK differ from those obtained by Hettich cytocentrifugation. In spite of the application of polycation-coated slides [2] mean cell recovery does not exceed 10% (range 2-15%) [3]. "Normal" CSF contains approximately 55% lymphocytes and approximately 45% monocytes. At high pleocytosis the difference between the two methods is lower. At normal cell count it is less probable to detect single "activated" B cells and plasma cells in sedimentation chamber preparations. However, by this technique large "erythrophages" are presented in good quality thereby enabling detection of _in vivo_ erythrocyte phagocytosis at a high rate.

The results point to advantages and disadvantages of Hettich cytocentrifugation and sedimentation of CSF cells and confirm the dependency of outcome of CSF cell examination on preparation techniques.

1. Lehmitz R (1991) Methoden zur Anreicherung von Liquorzellen. Lab Med 15: 41-45
2. Lehmitz R (1987) Verwendung von Polykationen-beschichteten Objektträgern für Zellanreicherungsverfahren. Z Med Lab Diagn 28: 222-224
3. Lehmitz R (1989) Liquorzellanreicherung mit der Sedimentkammer unter Verwendung von Polykationen-beschichteten Objektträgern. Psychiat Neurol Med Psychol 41: 751-754

Author index (page numbers)